The Ultimate Ride

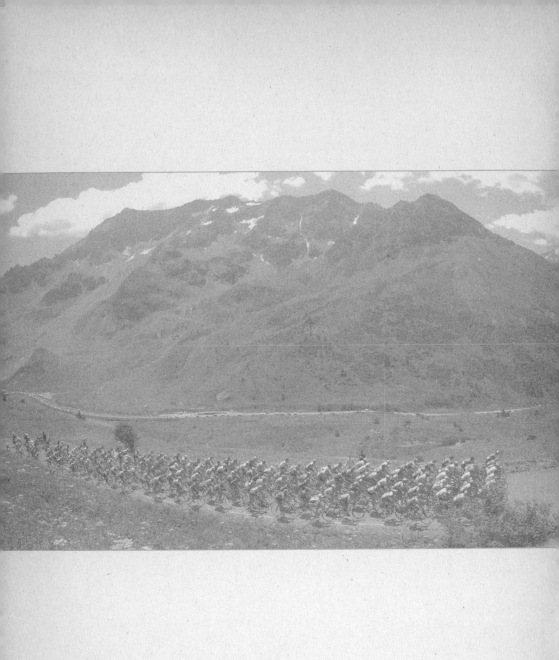

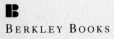

Berkley Books

The Ultimate Ride

Get Fit, Get Fast, and
Start Winning
with the
World's Top
Cycling Coach

Chris Carmichael

with Jim Rutberg

B

A Berkley Book
Published by The Berkley Publishing Group
A division of Penguin Group (USA) Inc.
375 Hudson Street
New York, New York 10014

This Book is an original publication of The Berkley Publishing Group.

While the authors have made every effort to provide accurate telephone numbers and Internet addresses at the time of publication, neither the publisher nor the authors assume any responsibility for errors, or for changes that occur after publication.

Penguin Group (USA) Inc. is not associated with Carmichael Training Systems, Inc., which is solely responsible for the information, services, and products offered herein.

CTS, FastPedal, Stomps, Flatsprints, Tempo, PowerInterval, HighSpeedSprint, PowerStart, OneLeggedPedaling, HillSprint, SpeedAccelerations, OverUnder, MuscleTension Intervals, ClimbingRepeats, HillAccelerations, DescendingIntervals, SpeedIntervals, SteadyState, PeakingProcess, EnduranceMiles, FixedGear, FoundationMiles, RaceSimulation, and RecoveryRate are trademarks or service marks of Carmichael Training Systems, Inc. The workout programs identified within this book are copyrighted works of CTS, Inc. No reproduction of this material is permitted without the express written permission of Carmichael Training Systems, Inc.

Spinning® is a registered trademark of Mad Dogg Athletics, Inc.

Copyright © 2003 by Carmichael Training Systems, Inc.
Book design by Amanda Dewey.

First Putnam hardcover edition: 2003
First Berkley trade paperback edition: June 2004
ISBN: 0-425-19601-1
Visit our website at www.penguin.com

Library of Congress Cataloging-in-Publication Data

Carmichael, Chris, date.
    The ultimate ride: get fit, get fast, and start winning with the world's top cycling coach / Chris Carmichael with Jim Rutberg. ·
        p. cm.
    ISBN 0-399-15071-4
    1. Bicycle racing—Training.   2. Physical fitness.   I. Rutberg, Jim.   II. Title.
GV1048.C39   2003   2003043214
    796.6'2—dc21

Printed in the United States of America
10 9 8 7 6 5 4 3 2

To Ed Burke,

whose knowledge was surpassed only by his humanity

Contents

Introduction

THE FIRST TIME I met Chris Carmichael, there was one big question I wanted to ask. It was the spring of 1999, a few months before Lance Armstrong's first Tour de France victory and the founding of Carmichael Training Systems. Chris had been my coach since the beginning of the year, but it was April before I met him on a trip to Colorado. He invited me up to his house for dinner, and within five minutes of stepping through his front door I asked, "Does a great coach produce great athletes, or is it the athletes that make the coach great?"

You see, Chris had only been my coach for a few months, and I was riding well, but not that much better than I would have been anyway. Besides his reputation, I didn't have any real proof that Chris was a great coach. Sure, he was Lance's coach, George Hincapie had introduced us, and he had coached the U.S. Olympic team, but the question still stood: Would those athletes have been just as successful regardless of whom they called "Coach"? Did Chris help them become great athletes, or did their greatness elevate Chris's coaching reputation just by association?

My question stopped Chris in his tracks: actually, it seemed like the whole house froze, and he asked me if I realized I had just questioned the validity of his and all coaches' careers. Suddenly I realized that my seemingly academic question was profoundly insulting. I had inadvertently stripped coaching of its worth and accused him of exploiting the athletes he worked with to further his career. The evening was not going anywhere near the way I had planned it.

Chris poured us each a glass of wine and set about answering my question. He said athletes are like students and coaches are their teachers. A talented and intelligent student has the tools to learn but needs instruction and guidance to become a scholar. Likewise, athletes like Lance Armstrong have the talent and drive to excel in cycling, but they need the same instruction and guidance to become champions. Would Lance have been a great cyclist without Chris? Chris's answer was yes. Had Chris improved Lance's performance beyond what he would have been capable of by himself? Again his answer was yes.

In the months that followed, I began to see the benefits of working with Chris. There was nothing earth-shattering about the training program—it was a sound program based on periodization and the principles and components of training. It was the instruction and guidance he mentioned over wine and dinner that night that made the difference. Chris challenged me to change the way I approached racing and training. I lacked confidence in my ability to ride aggressively, go off the front, and challenge riders I perceived to be better than I was. He used many of the same ideas you'll find in this book to show me how to find the confidence I needed to succeed. In a few weeks, I went from the back of the field to standing on the podium, and it had nothing to do with a change in my fitness. Maybe there *was* something to this whole coaching thing. . . .

I interned at CTS in the fall of 1999 and have been working here ever since. I made the transition from athlete to coach, and some time later Chris told me his first impression had been that I was a talented athlete but was a "head case." I was surprised, because I had thought my fitness and skills were what needed help, not my approach to racing. He had seen that I had the strength and talent to succeed but that I didn't know how to make the most of them. In the end, I had achieved what

Chris always knew I was capable of. What he had done only dawned on me later, after I had been coaching for a while. It turns out that the art of coaching involves guiding athletes to discover, on their own, what the coach already knows.

For three years I have worked alongside an unparalleled group of endurance coaches: Dean Golich, Craig Griffin, Chris Carmichael, Jim Lehman, Mike Niederpruem, and Lance Watson. I've seen them guide athletes through the same transformation that Chris helped me through, and they taught me to do it, too. Yet through it all, the question I asked Chris that night at his house still churned in my head: Which comes first, the great athlete or the great coach? Who makes whom?

The complete answer is somewhere in the middle. Talented athletes and coaches exist independently of each other. The mark of a great coach is the ability to improve any athlete's level of performance, regardless of that athlete's starting point. And when you combine the strengths of a great coach with the talent and drive of a great athlete, you create legends.

—Jim Rutberg

1

From the Ground Up

LONG BEFORE I THOUGHT of cycling in terms of fitness or competition, riding my bike offered freedom and a fun way to get from here to there. Some of my best memories from early childhood are of riding with a buddy from my house in South Miami, Florida, to Biscayne Bay. It was just a three-mile cruise each way, but it was an adventure to cover what seemed like a lot of territory. As I grew up and became a competitive racer, I never lost the sense of freedom and adventure I first enjoyed. Cycling has taken me around the world, introduced me to incredible people, and helped me develop a career through which I can positively affect the lives of many others by helping them reach their dreams.

When I was growing up in southern Florida in the 1960s, I was lucky that there was a well-developed cycling community. The large numbers of Cuban immigrants had brought their love for cycling with them when they settled in Miami, and there were plenty of cycling clubs, group rides, and training races. One of the local events, the Tour of Coconut

Grove, was my first taste of competition. I entered the race for the first time at nine years of age. It was a 10-years-old-and-under criterium and although I didn't really know what I was doing, I had a lot of fun and ended up finishing third. At such a young age, getting a trophy was a great feeling and I was completely hooked on bike racing.

I started riding my bicycle everywhere, including back and forth to and from school. One afternoon when I was 12, I stopped at a local arcade on the way home from school, locked up my bike, and went in to play pinball. When I left the arcade to go home, I found that someone had stolen my bike. I was particularly upset because I had convinced my parents to buy me a $90 bike and now I had lost it. Dade Cycle Shop was right next to the arcade, and I immediately went into the shop and asked for a job. I wanted to be able to go home and tell my dad I had lost my bike, but that I'd also gotten a job to pay for a new one.

Dade Cycle Shop was a racer's bike shop; they had Colnago bicycles hanging in the racks and racers working as mechanics. There wasn't much I knew how to do, but the owner, Joe Avalos, gave me a job after school fixing flat tires and sweeping up around the place. He had a couple of conditions for employing me. He told me not to talk too much and that if he found out my grades were suffering he would fire me. I think my starting salary was $1 an hour. Since I was the youngest person hanging around the shop, I quickly earned the nickname "The Kid," which has stuck with me to this day. Lance Armstrong still begins a conversation with me by saying, "Hey, Kid, how's it goin'?"

I learned a lot at Dade Cycle Shop, especially when I started going on training rides with the guys who worked there. I was several years younger than they were, and I had to learn quickly to draft well and ride intelligently to stay up with them. They also took the time to teach me basic racing skills, and about hydration and nutrition. I learned a lot of lessons the hard way: training in the afternoon without eating lunch, bonking far away from home, and finding myself in the middle of nowhere with a flat tire and no tools. But over time I improved as a cyclist and started placing consistently near the top of junior races. I guess I was about 16 when I realized I had some talent as a bike racer and decided to focus more attention on training for and winning races.

Many people helped me become a good amateur and, later, a professional cyclist, and their influences also helped shape my ideas around coaching and developing athletes. The people I met at Dade Cycle Shop—Joe Avalos, Bill Woodul, and Doug Martin—helped me learn about the sport, its history, heroes, and traditions. Doug was a mechanic and local racer, and years later we worked together when he was the U.S. Olympic Mountain Bike Team coach for the 1996 Olympics. David Ware was a racer in the Miami area who had taken an interest in coaching juniors. He wasn't that much older than I was, but he was an accomplished racer with the ability to teach. Later, when I got involved with the U.S. National Team and professional cycling, Eddy Borysewicz, Mike Neel, and Jim Ochowicz played large roles in helping me meet the demands of international competition.

My father and brother were very supportive and taught me the value of hard work and determination. Medical school runs in my family, and as the youngest child I seemed naturally headed in that direction. When I chose cycling instead of medicine, they were still supportive, but made it known I would have to make my own way. I decided to travel to pursue my goals in cycling, and in the late '70s there were two places to go to get into the big races: the Northeast and California. I couldn't afford to get to California, so I concentrated on the East Coast.

Dave Ware and I traveled around the East Coast, racing as often as we could. Dave was already a national-level racer, and I was getting there. Life had its fair share of ups and downs in those days: money was tight, the races were difficult, and good results were sporadic at best. Fortunately, the people around us were grounded and nurturing. Dave and I rode for the Stowe Bike Club, an established club in Vermont run by Jack Nash and other supportive and devoted cyclists. They made the rough times a little easier and helped us with food, clothes, equipment, and places to stay. Amateur cycling in the U.S. was, as it continues to be, a difficult environment to thrive in. There is very little consistency in the lifestyle of a full-time amateur cyclist, and it helps to surround yourself with good people who understand your goals and the passion you have for accomplishing them. Their ability to see the big picture as you struggle with details helps keep you on track. As it had in Florida, persistence paid off and it wasn't too long before my results started to consistently creep into the top ten.

Starting to ride for the U.S. Junior National Team was a big step for me. I believed in my abilities as a bike racer, but it was a huge boost to my confidence for the National Team coaches to say they wanted me to represent the United States in international competition. Competing with the National Team was also my first introduction to Eddy Borysewicz (Eddy B.). Before being involved in the National Team program, my training had very little structure. I did what most novice and intermediate cyclists still do; I rode hard when I

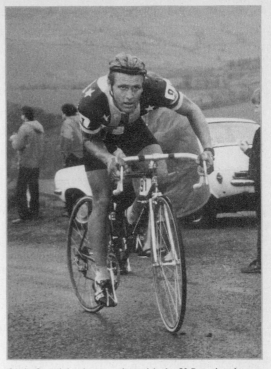

Chris Carmichael competing with the U.S. national team in the 1983 Milk Race in Ireland. Chris was a member of the National Team from 1978 to 1984. *Courtesy of Chris Carmichael*

felt good, rode as many hours as I could, and resisted taking time off.

The 1978 Junior World Championships was my first real experience with elite-level international competition. The race went reasonably well, but I realized there was a big difference between racing in the States and in Europe. These guys were tough, determined, and extremely fit. I realized that training in Europe was the only way to become competitive on the international level, and I moved to Holland to race for an amateur team called Gazelle in 1979.

Racing for the U.S. National Team had given me a few chances to experience international competition, but nothing prepared me for jumping headlong into Dutch, French, and Belgian amateur races. Instead of the support of the National Team and a peloton that accepted the presence of an American team, I was completely alone in a peloton that understood neither what I was doing there nor anything I said. I learned little bits of Dutch, Flemish, German, French, and Italian, none of which was suitable for polite company. And in the spirit of cultural exchange, I taught the peloton as many English expletives and insults as I could come up with.

I wasn't completely alone in Europe. The Kiwis, Aussies, and Canadians began arriving in Europe about the same time I did, as well as a small group of other Americans. Cycling was a European sport back then and it still is today. We were all outsiders, invaders of a sort, and we had to prove our right to stay. The racing and lifestyle were difficult, but I think we all felt a pioneer's pride that sustained us through the worst of it. I wanted to conquer the world, and every racer and director who cursed my presence strengthened my resolve to stay and succeed.

Well, I succeeded in staying in Europe, reaching the Olympic and professional levels of cycling, and holding my own against some of the best racers of the time, but I never quite managed to conquer the world. In December of 1986, I broke my femur while backcountry skiing in California. It was a bad break; I split my femur right up the center, starting at the knee, and there was a second fracture farther up. I had surgery and spent a long time in rehab, but I managed to return to the peloton for some of the 1987 season with 7-Eleven.

I learned a lot about the science of training in the process of coming back from my third knee surgery in as many years. It was really the first time in my cycling career that I had to find a creative way around an obstacle that hindered my performance. Dr. Edmund Burke, whom I had become friends with through the U.S. National Team, was instrumental in teaching me physiology so I could figure out how to manipulate my training to achieve the results I wanted. Other athletes started asking me questions about training and recovering from injuries, and I discovered that people understood things the way I explained them. One of Ed Burke's greatest gifts, and one of the most important lessons he taught me, was speaking about complicated concepts of physiology in ways everyone can comprehend and apply.

After my initial injury and two subsequent knee surgeries, I decided that 1989 would be my last year as a professional cyclist. I raced domestically that year for the Schwinn-Wheaties team, and although I could still win races, I knew I had lost something. Racing wasn't as fulfilling as it had been before, and though I got close, I could never quite regain top form. I retired at the end of the season and wondered what to do next.

Jiri Mainus helped make up my mind when he called and asked if I wanted to help out coaching some USA Cycling junior development camps. I enjoyed coaching immediately and realized I had an aptitude for it. The first group of racers I started working with included Lance Armstrong, George Hincapie, Bobby Julich, and Chann McRae. They were obviously strong and talented young riders, and I knew from my experiences at their age that the best thing I could do for their development was to take them to Europe.

Over the next few years, this ragtag group of teenagers made the transition from green amateurs to proficient professionals. They performed above everyone's expectations at the 1990 Amateur World Championships in Japan. In 1991, I put together an extensive program in Italy because I believed it was the best place to teach athletes how to succeed in Europe. At 19 years old, Lance won the Settimana Ciclistica Bergamasca, an important pro-am stage race in Italy. That victory, plus the performances of young athletes like Darren Baker and Steve Larsen, informed people that there was a group of young American stars on the horizon. The following year, the U.S. team campaigned in Spain prior to the Olympics in Barcelona and crushed the competition. We had extremely high hopes for the 1992 Olympics, but my final preparation schedule for the Games did not produce the results we were looking for. The guys weren't as fresh and sharp as I hoped they would be. Add to that losing Dave Nicholson from the team-time-trial squad due to a broken leg sustained while warming up, and my first Olympics as a coach didn't go as well as I'd hoped.

In the years leading up to the 1996 Olympics in Atlanta, Georgia, cycling in the United States took large steps forward with Project '96. The project's mission was to deliver the best technically, psychologically, and physically prepared athletes to Atlanta. We focused primarily on track disciplines because there are more medals available on the velodrome, and in timed track events like the one-kilometer time trial, individual pursuit, and team pursuit, where the strongest and best-prepared athletes win. I was appointed the Project's leader and expanded the coaching department by 300 percent, bringing it up to 18 full-time coaches, and hired two full-time sports scientists. I also recruited Dr. Edmund Burke to be Coordinator of Sport Science Services and Dr. Chester Kyle to be Bicycle Design Coordinator.

We had gained an enormous amount of knowledge between 1992 and 1996. The most visible advancement was in aerodynamics, culminating in the development of the GT Superbikes. But it takes more than slick bikes to win medals, and that's why I invested so heavily in coaches and sports scientists. We broke new ground in the science of endurance training, sports drinks, thermal regulation, altitude training, and the monitoring of athletic progress. The U.S. track-cycling program had two of its most successful years ever in 1994 and 1995. The athletes won five medals at the 1994 Track World Championships, part of the eight total medals that made up the all-time best medal count for a U.S. cycling team at the World Championships.

I continued to work as the head coach for USA Cycling through 1996, and decided after the Atlanta Olympics that I wanted to try something different. One of the things I had trouble with at USA Cycling was that we had developed a tremendous amount of information and knowledge, but it was only available to elite athletes in the National Team program. I thought we were under-delivering to the general membership. I knew I wanted to find a way to work with a broader scope of athletes and make quality coaching available to everyone, but I didn't know how I was going to do it.

THE FOUNDING OF CARMICHAEL TRAINING SYSTEMS

The next few years consisted of standing by Lance during his fight against cancer, consulting for various companies within the cycling and fitness industries, and picking up individual coaching clients. The combination was critical because Lance's comeback from cancer challenged me as a coach, the consulting work exposed me to many types of business models, and my individual clients helped me become more customer-oriented. The business model for Carmichael Training Systems (CTS) began to crystallize in the spring of 1999. With the help of my wife Paige and Simon Essl, Carmichael Training Systems was launched that September.

Two aspects of Carmichael Training Systems made me believe that we had solved the problem of disseminating world-class coaching information to the masses. The Internet offered the possibility of rapid communication between coach and athlete, as well as data storage and comparison. None of the athletes I was working with at the time, from Lance Armstrong and George Hincapie to my personal clients, lived in Colorado Springs. All the work I was doing was long-distance coaching, and though I could do it without the Internet, it was easier and faster on the Web. Economically it makes sense because, using the Internet, a single coach can work with enough athletes to make a living. That's an important consideration, because I firmly believe that CTS develops the best coaches by providing them the opportunity to make coaching a career. Career coaches are passionate about their jobs and don't have to split time between earning a living and doing what they love. And while the Internet made the business scalable, the lessons I learned during Lance Armstrong's comeback solidified the CTS coaching methodology.

Had I launched a company based on the coaching methodology I'd used with Lance prior to his cancer, the business would have failed in the first month. Lance's training was brutal, built on old-school theories that the best athletes are the ones who can survive the hardest workouts. You found an athlete's physiological limits, and pushed him over those limits until he either adapted or cracked. In the National Team program during the early 1990s, we burned through a lot of committed and talented cyclists using those theories; there was no way I was going to apply that methodology to cycling enthusiasts and amateur racers.

Following Lance's recovery from cancer, the old-school coaching methods didn't work for him anymore either. His body and his psyche couldn't withstand half the pressure they could before several surgeries and rounds of chemotherapy. So I went back to the basics of physiology to find a creative way around an obstacle, just as I had with my broken leg. Only this was much more than a broken leg; the battles he had waged against cancer ravaged his entire body. And besides atrophied muscles and a severely weakened aerobic system, Lance was dealing with survivorship issues; he was afraid that hard training might bring the cancer back, and he wasn't sure the sacrifices of professional cycling were worth the rewards. Restarting Lance's cycling career, and his passion for the sport, caused a huge shift in my coaching methodology.

I needed to figure out how to increase the precision of training, because the overall stress of his pre-cancer training program was too much for him. I sought to determine the limiting factor for endurance performance. What makes one athlete able to ride farther and faster than another?

Oxygen delivery to working muscles is the limiting factor for endurance performance, which means the aerobic system needs to be the cornerstone of endurance training. I started isolating Lance's workouts to his aerobic system, and the results were rapid and outstanding. Since the intensity was reduced, he could handle the workouts and recover from them quickly. The training wasn't as psychologically taxing either, so he maintained a positive outlook and improved his fitness at the same time. As his aerobic system increased in strength, his performance at higher intensities also improved, even though we hadn't been training at high intensities. A powerful aerobic engine improved anaerobic performance without the detrimental effects of training above lactate threshold. Now we're onto something. . . .

And so, CTS began with a new coaching methodology based on less pain and more gain. I contacted a few coaches I already knew and asked them if they would come work for me. I started writing about this new training methodology in the process of teaching coaches how to implement it, which led to training manuals for educating coaches and separate manuals for educating athletes.

Several of the coaches who worked on Project '96 now work for Carmichael Training Systems, including Craig Griffin, Mike Niederpruem, and Dean Golich. Griffin was the endurance track coach from 1990 to 2000, and he did a great deal of work applying new sports science research to altitude training and supplemental-oxygen training. Before the 1994 Track World Championships in Palermo, Italy, Griffin had his team-pursuit team on stationary trainers inside USA Swimming's flume. The environment in the flume could be programmed to simulate Palermo's humidity and elevation, allowing the athletes to live at altitude and train at and below sea level. Mike Niederpruem helped develop the coaching education program used to train USA Cycling coaches, and he has been instrumental in the coaching education program that CTS uses to train our coaches. Dean Golich was a sports scientist during Project '96, working with power meters and developing training protocols for the new Olympic mountain-bike team. I sought experts when CTS was in its infancy, because I wanted the best coaches to help train new coaches as the company grew. We trained more coaches, who in turn worked with more athletes, and the wealth of information these people possessed help me refine my ideas about coaching and put them into this book.

It has been said that the best coaches are not always the best competitors, and there is some truth to that statement. At the elite level, there are talented athletes and gifted athletes. Gifted athletes naturally excel early in their careers, but as you progress in racing, you have to work harder to continue to be successful. Eventually, the gift isn't enough anymore. Talented athletes can be as successful as gifted athletes, but they have to work harder from the beginning. When you find a gifted athlete who is willing to work as hard as a talented racer, you have the makings of a great champion. Lance Armstrong and Miguel Indurain are examples of gifted athletes whose incredible work ethics elevated them to the level of great champions. I believe I fall into the category of a talented cyclist who makes a better coach because of the amount of work I did in order to achieve my best performances. I had to learn the ins and outs of training, and search for ways to get just a little bit stronger.

Looking back on my 32 years of involvement in cycling, I am proud of my achievements as an athlete, but I believe I have accomplished more as a coach. My cycling career taught me that to achieve anything great, you have to take a great risk. I was part of the early wave of American cyclists to hit European shores, and there were no assurances that we would be successful at all. I learned through racing that you cannot experience success without first taking an equal amount of risk. And those lessons govern the way I live my life and run my business. When people see the Carmichael Training Systems logo, I want them to associate it immediately with the very best, tried-and-proven coaching service for the achievement of goals. I believe the coaching methodology I originally devised for endurance cycling can be successfully applied to any sport, to business, and to education. There are many risks inherent in pursuing my goals, but the goals are valuable enough to me to make the risks worth taking.

HOW TO USE THIS BOOK

Writing this book provided me with another way to fulfill the goal I left USA Cycling to pursue: to bring world-class coaching knowledge to athletes of all ability and experience levels. Whether you started cycling this week or have been racing for the majority of your life, I am confident that you will find this book informative, relevant, and useful. The book is designed around the CTS Pyramid of Success™, which illustrates the training methodology I developed through the course of Lance Armstrong's comeback from cancer. The material in the book is presented in roughly chronological order from the beginning of your cycling season through the completion of your goal event and end of your competitive season. As with actual training, it is important to learn the broadest concepts before working on details. The most important thing to realize is that all parts of this book, and all parts of your training, are interconnected. Nutrition and psychology are as important to your development as are your workouts.

I recommend reading this book cover to cover before beginning your training, and then referring back to it frequently during the year. A complete read should provide an overall picture about the ways your training in the beginning of the year will affect your performance during your goal event. There are examples of training blocks included in the book to guide you as you develop your program. Referring back to the text will help improve the effectiveness of your training during the individual periods of the year.

I've included a lot of information about racing tactics, and I believe that these tips are useful for competitors and noncompetitive athletes alike. Drafting, bridging gaps, warming up, eating right, and dressing properly are skills all cyclists need to understand. These things make cycling more efficient and enjoyable, and they improve your ability to perform at your best. I am a coach because helping you achieve your goals is what I find most fulfilling. If the information in this book helps you to reach a higher level of performance, then I have done my job.

This book contains a lot of useful information about the design and implementation of training, as well as my beliefs about properly preparing yourself for your ultimate ride. But regardless of how much information I write in books, there's no replacement for working one-on-one with a coach.

THE CTS PYRAMID OF SUCCESS™

The Pyramid of Success is the model that CTS coaches use to implement the coaching methodology I developed through my work with Lance Armstrong. The Pyramid of Success hanging on the wall in my office looks like this:

100% Ready

Peaking Process

Specialization * Confidence

Nutritional Plan * Pre, Post, During

Preparation Training * Skill Development

Aerobic Strength * Foundation and Resistance Training

Energy Systems * Components and Principles of Training * Periodization

Goal Setting * Psychological Fitness * Imagery * Stress Management * Mental Drills™

Pyramid of Success: Level 1 (Chapter 2)

The whole process of reaching peak performance begins with determining what you want to achieve and preparing yourself for the challenges that lie ahead. I place extreme importance on your goals, attitude, and mental fortitude, because there is no escaping the difficulty of achieving peak performance. Your goals have to be appropriate to your initial skill and fitness level, valuable to you, and realistic yet challenging.

Pyramid of Success: Level 2 (Chapter 3)

The second level of the Pyramid builds upon that foundation. Understanding how your body's energy systems function and adapt to training is critical, because you are going to use this information to determine the types of training needed to improve your fitness. You need to understand principles and components of training. Your training success is achieved through manipulating these variables. Finally, the application of periodization (the process of breaking the training year into smaller, focused segments) defines the timeline upon which your performance progresses. You have to start with a goal, and then work backward along the timeline to establish the length and placement of individual training segments. Your goals establish when you have to be 100% Ready, and this level of the Pyramid of Success elevates you to where you can begin to achieve your goals.

Pyramid of Success: Level 3 (Chapter 4, Chapter 5)

Physical training begins in the third level of the Pyramid, and this illustrates that conditioning is only a part of what makes an athlete successful. Beginning training without first establishing goals and a plan for achieving them is like setting sail without a compass, map, or sextant. The aerobic system is the limiting factor for endurance performance, so your success is dependent on building the strongest aerobic engine you can. The upper levels of the Pyramid will collapse under their own weight unless your aerobic and strength training develop an indestructible foundation to support them.

Pyramid of Success: Level 4 (Chapter 6)

The fourth level of the Pyramid is where your aerobic foundation begins to improve your ability to handle higher intensities. While still working to develop your aerobic engine, you will add workouts at your maximum sustainable workload. Because of the work you did strengthening your aerobic system, you will be able to sustain a higher workload while relying on your anaerobic energy system for a lower proportion of the energy. This means you will be able to work out longer before fatigue sets in, and you will make more significant fitness gains. Skill development is included in this level of the Pyramid because you will probably be participating in group training sessions or early-season competitions at this time. Success in cycling is based as much on skill as on fitness, so it is important to learn *how* to perform well, so you know what to do as a 100% Ready Athlete™.

Pyramid of Success: Level 5 (Chapter 7)

I could have placed nutrition at the same level as goal-setting and mental preparation, because I believe it is one of the most important factors in optimal performance. It is the fifth level of the Pyramid because the fuel you put in your body becomes more critical the closer you get to being 100% Ready. What you eat affects the quality of your workouts, your ability to recover between them, your ability to build and repair muscle, and your body weight. Your dietary requirements change as you move through the training year and need to be monitored and adjusted frequently.

Pyramid of Success: Level 6 (Chapter 8)

Specialization is the sixth level of the Pyramid of Success, and this is the turning point of your season. If you have been keeping up with your training, achieving your smaller goals, and maintaining your focus, the Specialization level of the Pyramid provides the boost you need to elevate your performance to an optimal level. The reason that this is a turning point for your season is that the high training intensity of this level will expose any weaknesses in your preparation to this point. Everything you have done so far has been aimed at providing the strength required to support this level.

Pyramid of Success: Level 7 (Chapter 9)

The Peaking Process is the final step to becoming 100% Ready, and it is as simple as it is complex. The goal of the peaking process is to deliver you to your goal event rested, motivated, primed, and sharp. Timing is of great importance, because your goal is to be at your best on the day of your goal event.

Pyramid of Success: Level 8 (Chapter 10)

The 100% Ready Athlete™ possesses fitness, confidence, and total preparedness. Your fitness has developed through the planned steps of your training program, and your confidence has grown as a result of achieving the training goals for which you have prepared. Your success as a 100% Ready Athlete™ does not hinge on victory, but rather on your ability to compete at the best of your ability.

One of the reasons I use a pyramid to model the CTS coaching methodology is that its shape illustrates the idea that your focus narrows as you approach your goal event. The lower levels of the Pyramid are strong, but they're broad. As you move up the Pyramid, your goals and workouts become more detailed, so by the time you are 100% Ready, you have a firm grasp on every detail of optimal performance. In the beginning of the year, there's a lot of room to make modifications and plenty of time to get back on track if you get distracted. But as time goes by, it becomes increasingly important that you stay on track, because there isn't enough time to regain the path and still make it to your destination on time.

THE NEED FOR A COACH

A coach is an essential part of achieving athletic success, and the continued successes of CTS members confirm that. Coaching puts a human touch on the science and regimen normally associated with training, molding it to the individual demands and limitations we all face. Lance's best-selling book is titled *It's Not About the Bike*, and when I started this project I jokingly wanted to call it *It's Not About the Training Program*. It's a corny title, but it illustrates an important point. Lance's successes, and the successes of all the athletes CTS works with, are due to more than just great training programs. Prescribing training is only one of the jobs coaches do every day, because a training program is just a road map, or in our case, a pyramid. I communicate with Lance Armstrong almost every day of the year, because he and I know there's more to winning the Tour de France than performing a specific workout on a specific day. Coaching is about inspiring and motivating athletes to achieve goals they find valuable, and about improving the sense of fulfillment and enjoyment a person gets from life. My best days as a coach aren't necessarily when athletes win competitions, but rather when I have helped someone make a positive change in his or her life.

Athletes coached by CTS have the option of filling out monthly member reports, which I read and use to ensure that CTS coaches are helping people achieve their goals. I have saved some of them and would like to share a few:

Byron Taylor is a 59-year-old engineer who started working with CTS coach Jim Lehman in 2001.

> My training and relationship with my CTS coach have benefits beyond cycling. Through periods of great personal and professional stress, my coach has coped with my endless complaints about everything from the weather to back pains. But my daily routine of scheduled, structured workouts allows me to start my days with a feeling of accomplishment and satisfaction. No matter what happens later in the day, I know I have already completed something positive.

Blair Mathieson is a mountain-bike racer who is coached by CTS coach James Herrera and who overcame some initial skepticism to have a very successful racing season:

> The CTS philosophy of "Less Pain, More Gain" was the most counter-intuitive point I'd ever heard of. I always thought I had to go as fast as possible in training, so that my body could better handle racing speed. So naturally when I joined CTS, I fought with my coach about building slow, "easy" endurance miles. I couldn't understand how going slower, with "less pain," was going to help me go faster at higher pain levels. It didn't make any sense. Then I raced after six months of these "easy miles" and it was amazing. I rode the entire race faster then I've ever gone, at lower heart-rate levels, and my thinking about training changed 180 degrees. I consider myself a "born again" CTS member.

Steve Reker worked with CTS coach Ryan Oelkers to return to competition after being hit by a car while training:

My coach has been a big help with the mental aspects of training. Bad days and poor races are now part of the program and things to learn from, not things to stay depressed about. The positive encouragement from my coach goes a long way to keeping me going during a long season.

Janice Tower is one of my favorite CTS members. She lives and trains in Alaska for ultra-endurance events, and, working with CTS coach Jane Beezer, she balances training with raising a family and having a career:

At age 38 I decided to take on two challenges that begged to be met: the 100-mile Iditasport winter mountain-bike race in Alaska, and the 24 Hours of Moab. As a working mother of two kids, I knew that a training program would have to make efficient use of my time. I think I told my coach, Jane Beezer, "I just want to see how far I can take this thing!" Not only was my training program designed to suit my lifestyle, but the concepts of periodization and focused training effort gave me the most benefit for the time I had available. Since signing on with CTS in 2000, I've competed in two 24-Hour World Championships, finishing as high as 4th place, and I have become the third woman to finish the 350-mile Iditarod Trail Invitational, a winter mountain-bike race from Anchorage to McGrath, Alaska. Each year seems to build on the previous years' successes, and I look forward to many more years of fun as a CTS athlete.

You are more likely to stay involved in an exercise program if you are working with a coach. There's someone there to hold you accountable for the things you said you wanted to do. A coach provides the personal guidance and expertise to integrate your training into your lifestyle so you can achieve your goals without sacrificing your relationships or career. By minimizing the obstacles between you and your goals, a coach improves your chances for success and makes the process of succeeding more enjoyable.

Athletes of all ability levels benefit from working with a coach, and novice athletes can benefit most of all. Success as an endurance athlete depends heavily on the skills and habits you develop early in your participation in the sport. Endurance training is cumulative over a period of several years, and starting that process correctly helps you progress more rapidly.

Barry Norman wrote the following after his first Assault on Mount Mitchell ride, and the next year he took an hour off his time for the same event:

> I first started riding a bicycle because every other member of my family was athletic. My wife and her brothers and sisters were all runners and triathletes, and though they didn't pressure me to exercise, I wanted to fit in with the family a little better. I was overweight, out of shape, and hadn't exercised much since high school. My first ride was three miles around my neighborhood and I was sore for days. I kept riding and steadily improved, but I didn't like the ambiguity of not knowing what I was doing. My brother is a cyclist and he planned on riding an event called the Assault on Mount Mitchell. It is a 103-mile ride in North Carolina that finishes with a 30-mile climb up Mount Mitchell. In December I set a goal of completing the ride the following June, and decided I needed professional help to prepare. My CTS coach, Josh Seldman, designed a training program that met the demands of the event (11,000 total feet of climbing) and my schedule (8 to 10 hours/week). I was shocked that his training schedule was so easy; it didn't have nearly as many hard workouts as I had been doing previously. By June, I was a changed man. I had dropped 20 pounds and learned about eating and drinking on the bike. The Assault on Mount Mitchell was the longest ride I have ever done, and I had to stop several times, but I made it to the finish line in eight hours and forty-one minutes. I never would have made it without Josh's guidance, and as I hugged my wife I decided I wanted Josh to help me finish the Assault faster next year.

Purchasing this book makes you eligible to try CTS coaching for free. I am offering this promotion to you because I want to give you the opportunity to experience working with a coach. For many of you, high school was the last time you worked with a coach, and you may be skeptical about a CTS coach's ability to help you. In the first three years that CTS has been in business, our high member-retention rates have set new standards for the industry. The vast majority of people who try CTS coaching find it valuable enough to stick with it, which is why I am confident you'll see the benefits of coaching when you try it too.

2

Foundation for Success:
Your Mental Preparation
for Achievement

WHAT SEPARATES TALENTED ATHLETES from champions? Oftentimes, the answer lies in the way they approach training and competition. Those who approach cycling as a solely athletic challenge often fall short of their true potential. True champions, on the other hand, understand that realizing their potential requires a holistic approach to success. Athletic success results from training the mind and body to work as one. Mental training is as critical to achievement as physical training, and an athlete's mental approach to training and competition often makes the difference between standing on the top step of the podium and watching the awards ceremony from a distance.

Sports psychology is important, because you have to be mentally prepared for the demands of training and competition. There are some aspects of cycling that are predictable: you will have to put in many hours of hard training, you will have to deal with the lonely nature of training, you will have to deal with high levels of sustained intensity, and you will have to remain focused and motivated through the duration of a long season. There are also aspects of this sport that you cannot control: the weather and your equipment will not always cooperate, crashes will happen, and other obligations will put constraints on your time.

Mental training helps you deal with both the predictable and the unpredictable challenges you will inevitably face. The best athletes I have had the honor to work with are well-rounded individuals. They are committed to their athletic goals, they train hard, and they keep a healthy perspective of the role cycling plays in their lives.

Training is a matter of balance. You have to balance the physical and psychological loads with adequate rest and time away from the regimen of training. A well-structured training program applies a load that stresses your body to lead to positive adaptation. A well-developed set of mental skills provides you with the resources to make the most of the physical prowess you are creating.

THE SIX MISCONCEPTIONS OF MENTAL TRAINING

Before we get into the details of your mental preparation for success, let's dispel some common misconceptions about mental training:

1. *Mental skills training can make up for physical weaknesses.*
   If the rider next to you is in better shape than you are, and if he used some mental skills training too, he will beat you. Being mentally prepared for competition is beneficial, but there are no shortcuts to winning bike races. Mental training is not an excuse to do less physical training; it is an addition that makes your total training program more complete.

2. *Mental skills training is only for elite athletes.*
   One of the main reasons I founded Carmichael Training Systems is that I believed that athletes of all levels should be able to benefit from the same quality of coaching that elite athletes receive. A key component of that belief is that the training and coaching techniques I use are equally applicable to Lance Armstrong and you.

The same skills that allow an elite athlete to excel at high levels can help beginners learn skills more efficiently, and thus help them reach their full potential more quickly and effectively.

3. *Mental skills training can provide a quick fix needed for success at an important competition.*
Unfortunately, there is no quick fix involved in mental skills training. Mental skills are precisely that: skills. As with physical or technical skills, individuals are naturally talented in some areas and need practice in others. Mental skills need to be learned, coached, practiced, and reinforced in order to provide benefit.

4. *Mental skills training is not useful.*
Many people believe that mental skills training is not useful for athletes because it seems too "touchy-feely" or New Age. The Australian Olympic program's success in the 2000 Sydney Olympics supports the concept that sports psychology is beneficial for athletes.

With a population of only 19 million people, less than the population of California alone, Australia won 58 medals in the 2000 Olympics. They did not have the luxury of the immense talent pool available in the United States. In this country, there is an abundance of athletes with the talent to reach the Olympic Games. When one athlete succumbs to the pressure of competing at the elite level, several other athletes are prepared to take his or her place. The Australians often have only one or two athletes in each sport capable of competing at the Olympic level. As a result, the Australian Olympic Committee focuses on nurturing their smaller pool of elite athletes by concentrating on mental exercises and believing that athletes need to be both mentally and physically prepared for competition. Their work paid off, and Australia won more medals, per capita, than any nation in the 2000 Olympic Games.

5. *Mentally tough cyclists are born, not made.*
The Lance Armstrong you see today is the result of heredity and personal evolution. He is not the same man he was when he was

18 or 21 years old. His determination and commitment to his goals developed over time, along with his athletic potential. Mental skills training cannot make you a Tour de France champion if you don't have the physical capacity, but it can help you achieve your full potential.

6. *Good mental skills mean never feeling nervous.*
   All athletes get nervous at some point. It may be at the start line, the base of a huge climb, five kilometers from the finish, or lying in bed in the middle of the week. Nervousness and anxiety are normal human emotions, and eliminating them entirely is not the goal of mental skills training. Rather, you are trying to get a handle on your mental state so that you can control your anxiety, maybe even redirect your nervous energy to fuel your performance.

Mental skills training can have a number of beneficial effects on your performance: increased self-awareness, increased training consistency, increased self-confidence, and increased motivation.

FINE-TUNE YOUR MENTAL FITNESS

Fitness is built through working on broad-based concepts first, and then narrowing the scope of training to finer details. In physical training, we always start with base aerobic conditioning and end up with specific, detail-oriented workouts the closer we get to important races. The same is true for building mental fitness. There are three main factors that need to be considered when trying to achieve peak performance: Personality and Motivational Factors, Peak Performance Strategies, and Skills for Coping with Adversity. These factors can be thought of as sides of a triangle, with Personality and Motivational factors as the triangle's base. Peak Performance Strategies and Skills for Coping with Adversity are the detailed skills that you apply to your base of Personality and Motivational Factors.

I work with an athlete named Steve. Along with being a committed cyclist, he is also an investment banker with a wife and two small chil-

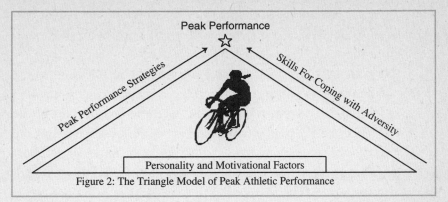

Figure 2: The Triangle Model of Peak Athletic Performance

Adapted from Gould, D. and Damarjian, N. (1998). Mental skills training in sport. In B. Elliot (Ed.). *Training in sport: Applying sport science* (pp. 69–116). Chichester, UK: John Wiley & Sons. Copyright © 1998 by John Wiley & Sons Limited. Reproduced with permission.

dren. The base of Steve's triangle for peak athletic performance is characterized by his personality. Steve is your standard Type-A personality: he is high-energy, uncompromising, highly motivated, and obstinate. He is a perfectionist who comes unglued when things go wrong.

Steve's strong sense of motivation and his perfectionist tendencies are good for his athletic endeavors. They ensure that he will be able to stick to the long hours of training and stay focused on the tasks at hand each day. But as we develop his physical engine to make him a more competitive athlete, we will also have to work on his inflexibility in adverse conditions. It is important for athletes to be able to overcome adversity and still put forth a superlative effort. We will have to develop performance strategies that enable Steve to balance his busy life with his commitment to training as well. The goal in fine-tuning his mental fitness is to let him achieve his athletic goals without sacrificing his family or working relationships.

CONFIDENCE: THE MOST IMPORTANT MENTAL SKILL

A successful athlete is a confident athlete. Of course, it's easy to be confident if you are already a successful athlete, if you are already winning races. The catch here is that you have to be self-confident before you have achieved athletic success. In a society in which we are taught that humility is preferable to pride, many people have trouble with self-confidence; they mistake confidence for boastfulness or cockiness.

If you plan on winning a bike race, you have to be able to go to the start line knowing that you are capable of beating every person standing with you. When Lance Armstrong puts his name on the start list of the Tour de France, he is essentially walking up to the best cyclists in the world and saying, "I am going to beat you. Not only am I going to beat you today, I am going to beat you day after day, and after 23 days I am going to win this race." The reason that this is confidence and not cockiness is that there are several other team leaders who are saying the same thing when they enter the race. If you want to win, you can't doubt your abilities. You can, and must, respect the abilities of the other competitors, but it is perfectly all right to think you are going to beat them. If you don't believe you are going to beat everyone, how do you expect to win the race?

How do you develop the confidence to know you can beat the racers around you, before you have actually proven you *can* win races? Confidence comes from success, and your brain doesn't necessarily care whether that success was in training or competition. In 1999, I started working with an athlete who was a capable rider in elite-level domestic races, but not a consistent top-ten finisher. As we got to know each other, I realized that because he had never beaten certain riders from several pro teams, he didn't believe he was strong enough to compete with them. His confidence was low because he was focusing on results, not on the process of achieving those results. So we started setting process goals for races. He focused on making the breakaways, staying in the top fifteen riders in the peloton, and riding aggressively. He quickly realized that he could ride aggressively and still finish races. He could attack the pros and make them hurt. Those experiences gave him the confidence to go to the start line with the knowledge that he could beat every man standing with him.

An underconfident athlete is tentative and conservative, and has higher levels of anxiety that undermine the ability to perform. Think about how you raced in your last big event. Did you initiate the attacks during the race, or did you always follow wheels? Were you hesitant to take a pull at the front because you feared being dropped? Did you back down when another rider challenged you for a position in the peloton? These are all signs of an underconfident competitor. Next time your brain doubts the ability of your legs and lungs to attack, take a pull, or take a wheel; override your initial reaction and go for it. Sometimes you will succeed and sometimes you won't, but you will only gain confidence by sticking your neck out and risking failure. The first coach I ever had pulled me aside following a junior criterium in Miami. I had let up well before the finish line and lost the final sprint. What he said to me stuck with me throughout my entire racing career: "You can't win if you don't sprint."

An overconfident athlete overestimates his abilities and is sometimes underprepared to put forth his best effort due to an inaccurate belief he is properly prepared. An example of this is an athlete who forgoes hill training because he always leads everyone to the summit of a climb in the Tuesday group ride. Believing that his climbing skills and fitness are so great that he doesn't need to train any more may lead to a rude awakening when he gets dropped on a large climb in a race. Between 1999 and 2002, Lance Armstrong won eight time trials in the Tour de France, but he never turned down the chance to train for time-trial efforts. He understands that the reason he wins time trials is due to the specific training he does; it is not because of an innate, naturally occurring talent for time trials.

Ideally, athletes need to have a healthy, realistic sense of their abilities and what they need to accomplish. A positive, healthy sense of self-confidence increases their abilities to concentrate, provides a positive mental state, and enhances the quality of their efforts. Use the following tips to help foster confidence in your abilities to reach peak performance:

1. Reflect on past successes to overcome natural feelings of self-doubt.
2. Focus on the things you can control: your training, preparation, and proactive racing strategies.
3. Avoid excessive worrying about what others expect from you (e.g., don't let pressure from teammates prevent you from racing aggressively).

4. Don't let perceived deficiencies in one area (climbing, for instance) imply that you are deficient in other areas (like sprinting).

5. Compete to achieve instead of competing to avoid failure.

6. In your daily training log, write down one positive thing about each and every training session. Review these positive notes to remind yourself of your accomplishments.

GOAL-SETTING

Everyone has the desire to do his or her best, to excel, to attain the highest standards of performance. I have seen firsthand the desire Lance Armstrong has for cycling excellence and how it has led him to reign supreme in his chosen field. Often the most difficult barriers you face in achieving success are those you impose upon yourself, sometimes unknowingly. Psychological barriers can become our toughest opponents and obstacles to achieving success. Success starts with a belief—a dream—that you can achieve. This dream gives birth to reality.

Perhaps the best example of how success starts with belief in yourself is Lance Armstrong's journey as an athlete. I have been Lance's personal coach since 1990, and we have developed quite a close relationship. Over time, this relationship has grown from a strict coach/athlete one to a close friendship based on mutual respect.

Diagnosed with cancer, Lance battled for his life. Throughout long and difficult bouts of chemotherapy, he still thought of racing successfully again at the international level. Without Lance's strong commitment to reaching his desired goals, he never would have come close to racing again.

Early in 1998, it appeared that Lance would limit his participation in stage races. At the time, it seemed that there were physical reasons why he wouldn't be successful in the day-after-day grind of stage racing. Accordingly, I devised a new racing plan and changed the way Lance played the game. During the months of March, April, and May, Lance raced less than a dozen times. This was not the tried-and-true approach, but in his first race back in Europe, he won! Lance focused on specific goals and was stage racing to greater success than he had ever achieved before his cancer. Before you can chase your dreams, you must know exactly what they are and where you are in relation to them. You must also have the courage to make your own rules and not allow yourself to be governed by perceived or imposed limitations.

Goals Require Commitment

Commitment to improving your performance is something you must establish for yourself. No one can tell you what is important in your life—that is your decision. It is clear that successful athletes are highly committed to excellence. There is no way to achieve a high level of excellence in your training without a high level of commitment. When the question "How important is your cycling success?" was posed to members of the U.S. National Cycling Team, it was clear that the most successful athletes from this already highly successful group were those who demonstrated the greatest commitment to cycling. These athletes were fueled by high-octane passion and dedication, and these values were simply a daily fact of their lives. The greater your commitment to training, the more your life will focus on achieving success. Lance Armstrong's commitment to success in cycling means that his life centers on eating, sleeping, and training. This level of commitment increases his chances of successful performances.

Even professional cyclists sometimes struggle with commitment. Back in 1996, Lance was a huge favorite for medals in the Atlanta Olympics. His season had unfolded beautifully, including a win in the Fleche-Wallone Classic, a strong second place in Liege-Bastogne-Liege, and his complete dominance of the Tour du Pont. He was committed to the goal of medaling at the Olympics, but there was something missing. It was not until after his recovery from cancer and his first Tour de France victory that I really realized what had been missing in 1996. Lance's Atlanta Olympic goal was important to him, but it was not his central focus. He was focused on being a successful professional cyclist, which at the time meant winning as many events as possible. He was committed to the Olympics, but he was equally committed to the World Cup, to the Tour du Pont, and to winning Classics. When he didn't perform up to his expectations in one event, he put it behind him without another thought and immediately turned his focus to the next race. He never dealt with the disappointment he felt over losing. He suppressed that disappointment by focusing on a new goal, and he didn't get too attached to any race.

After recovering from cancer and finishing fourth in the 1998 Tour of Spain, the Road World Championships, and the Time Trial World Championships, Lance was inspired to look seriously at competing in the Tour de France as a potential winner. For the first time, he committed his whole being to an event, and that event took on a great presence in his life. Previously, his partial commitment to individual races had resulted in his partial achievement of his potential. Lance's dominating performance in the 1999 Tour de France is the best example I can show for the power of commitment.

Matching Lance's commitment to training will most likely not be possible for you. Many of the daily duties of life limit us from having the luxury of devoting a majority of our time to training. There is a point at which we must measure our wish list against our daily duties. There is only so much time in a day, and it must be shared among work, family or relationship obligations, training, and rest. Realistically, we all have limits to our commitment to training, and for most of us those commitments change often. You must also consider the impact of training on others in your life and work to ensure their long-term support of your goals. Your dedication to training can dramatically affect your progress. Strong commitment assists in establishing crucial mental components such as desire, determination, passion, and self-motivation. These mental components will tilt the balance between "doing it" and "not doing it."

Goal-Setting—Putting It All Together

In cycling, outstanding performances involve the whole person: mind and body. Establishing goals is the first step in your preparation for success. The next step in mental preparation is to develop a strong strategy as to how you will achieve the goals.

Goals that provide direction for training activities are most helpful. With established goals, it is easier to determine when training gets off track so you can take action to regain control. Without goals, it is difficult to assess whether you are on track and making progress in your training.

It is essential that you take ownership of your goals. Coaches, family members, and teammates cannot make your goals for you. If you want to complete your first century (a 100-mile bike ride), win a Masters District Championships, or take a medal at Nationals, it has to be *your* goal, not the goal someone else established for you. When training gets difficult and your motivation takes a dive, someone else's goal is not going to provide the support and desire to let you continue. A goal that is yours, that you own, and that you value is going to get you out the door and keep you on track.

Be Specific

The more specific your goals, the more effectively they can positively direct your training. Broad, general goals are not reliable in directing training. Many times, long-term, far-off goals or dream goals do not focus enough energy on the present. CTS's coaching experience indicates that an athlete should use dream-term goals to motivate and stretch personal limits, but mid-term and micro-goals are essential for reaching the desired larger goal.

Stay in Control

There are many aspects to competition that are out of your control, including mechanical failures, competitors, and climate conditions. You will increase your opportunity for success when your energy is focused on the performance aspects of cycling that are within your control. I prefer to emphasize training goals rather than race results for short-term goals that measure progress. Your chances of achieving competitive success are greatly increased if you are in good condition and ready to race, so stay focused on what you can control: your training, conditioning, and workouts. Setting appropriate goals will always keep you on track and focused on the controllable aspects of performance. At times, athletes become embattled with outside factors and lose commitment to the very core aspects that create success. Stay in control and maintain focus.

CTS member Blair Mathieson provided an example of the benefit of basing goals on training progress rather than results in one of his member reports:

> My first major goal was to win the Sport Sea Otter Classic. Before that race, I had never won a Sport mountain-bike event. I trained religiously under the program, constantly harassing my coach about the lack of intensity in my training, even thinking about quitting the program at times. My coach kept me focused. His e-mail messages were personalized, lengthy replies. I didn't feel like I was just a "number," and many a time he lifted my spirits in the dead of winter when training can be such a bore. At the Sea Otter Classic, I ended up leading the race by a couple of minutes with a mile left, when I flatted just before the paved road started. Even though I didn't win, I knew that my fitness had increased tenfold.

I always design an athlete's training program by first reviewing established goals. I want to know what an athlete is going to be satisfied with accomplishing. Those goals provide valid and attainable measurements for success. Goals established by an athlete ensure that training is focused on developing the athlete's energy systems correctly. You need to ask yourself what you expect to achieve from your training program. Do you expect to improve speed, power, or endurance? You will find that your training goals help motivate you while training alone, creating a sense of personal satisfaction from the workouts. Your training program must reflect the goals you have established. It is difficult, if not impossible, for an athlete to reach the limits of his or her talent without using goals to design training programs.

DREAM GOALS

At the top end of the goal spectrum are dream goals, or ultimate goals that push the limits of possibility. Dream goals are the ones you have difficulty admitting to anyone except your closest friends. Talking about your dream goals can put you in an uncomfortable position. They are the goals that people may laugh at you for even considering. Dream goals

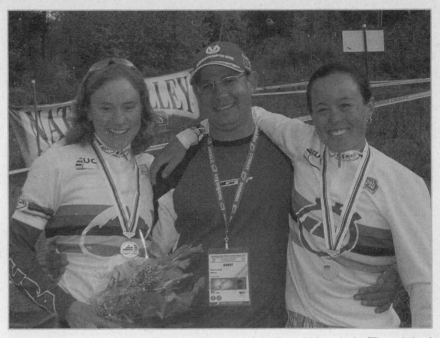

Alison Dunlap (left) and Mari Holden (right) set extremely ambitious goals. Through hard work and several years working with CTS coach Dean Golich (center), both earned World Championship titles. *Photo courtesy of Dean Golich*

seem worlds away when you set them, and they tend to be very inspiring. Many of the athletes I have worked with have been almost afraid to talk out loud about the goal they are ultimately shooting for because it seems too outlandish. Lance Armstrong was one such athlete. In 1990, he dreamed about winning the Tour de France, but he had a hard time openly admitting it. As a coach, part of my job is to bring those seemingly preposterous goals into the light, and to provide the support necessary to make an athlete truly believe that dreams are possible.

Set your dream goals high. One of my younger athletes wanted to go to the Olympics, and had since he was a little kid. After several years of racing and making steady progress, he was still far from achieving his goal of making the Olympic cycling team. The closest he came to the Olympics was an opportunity to race for the U.S. National Team in an international event. After retiring from racing a few years later, having never reached the Olympics, he told me he had no regrets about not making the team. He sent me an e-mail in which he said:

I decided early on to shoot for the stars, figuring that if I fell short, I would at least reach the moon. But had I been more conservative with my goals, and only tried to reach the moon, falling short would have left me in the middle of nowhere. In my mind, riding for the National Team was a necessary step to making the Olympic team. Keeping my eyes on the Olympic team took the pressure off the goal of making the National Team, thus making that goal more attainable. I have applied that same idea to the rest of the goals in my life, and so far it has yet to let me down.

Dream goals are goals that are long shots, but possible if everything falls into place. These goals can help you through tough times and also serve as food for fantasy on long rides. As with all goals, write down your dream goal and refer back to it regularly to remind yourself where you're going and what the ultimate prize is.

CONFIDENCE-BUILDING GOALS

Mid-term goals are often the end-points of a training cycle. They are a way of confirming the effectiveness of the training you have been doing in recent weeks or months. A mid-term goal focuses your efforts on achieving something realistic but ambitious. These goals are a crucial part of the performance evaluation process that helps you stay on track. Focusing on the primary goal of the season is too intimidating for most athletes. Confidence-building goals alleviate this pressure by breaking that primary goal into more manageable chunks. If winning the district criterium is your goal for the year, and the race is still ten months away, focusing on a confidence-building goal that is two months away ensures that you can maintain your commitment to training. Planning a series of ambitious goals along the way helps to define the path to success in your primary event. These goals also enable you to make necessary modifications to your training before it is too late.

Walker Ferguson's primary goal for 2001 was to win the U23 Mountain Bike World Championship. He had a precedent for his World Championship goals. In 2000, he had won the Junior Mountain Bike World

Championship and earned a pro contract with the Subaru Gary Fisher professional mountain-bike team. His 2001 training plan included a pretty heavy period of European road racing with the Under-23 (U23) national team. He returned to the U.S. in July to compete in a NORBA National event in Durango, Colorado—an event we had established as a confidence-building goal. He gave it everything he had and still did not perform very well. The event showed that with ten weeks to go before the World Championships, Walker was not where he needed to be, physically, to achieve his goal for the season. Evaluating his performance markers through testing and data collected from a powermeter on his bicycle, it was clear to me that he needed more work on his anaerobic power. He was having trouble handling the repeated bouts of maximal effort required in mountain-bike racing.

Walker was pretty discouraged after Durango, and it would have been easy for him to give up on his season goal. As an outside party, I was less discouraged. We had purposely set up his confidence-building goal

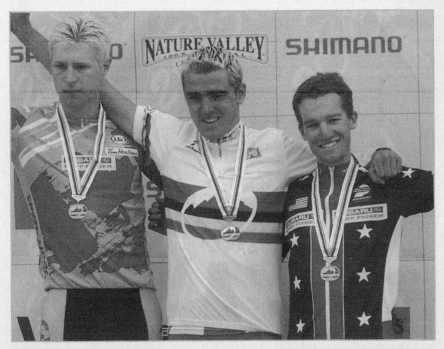

Walker Ferguson (right) smiling from the podium at the 2001 Mountain Bike World Championships. *Photo © by Simon Essl*

far enough ahead of his primary goal that we could modify his training and keep him on track for Worlds. In the end, the Durango race did exactly what it was meant to do: it allowed Walker and me to get a very honest evaluation of his performance and use that evaluation to direct his training. Ten weeks later, Walker won a bronze medal in the cross-country event at the 2001 Mountain Bike World Championships, in his first year in the U23 age group.

How do you determine what to use as an appropriate confidence-building goal? It should be an event where the physical and mental demands of the competition are similar to those in your primary goal. If you are aiming to win a medal at the Road National Championships, a strong performance in a large regional road race makes a good confidence-building goal. Remember that you will be competing in a confidence-building race in less-than-peak condition, since you are aiming to be in peak condition for your primary goal. With this in mind, the difficulty of the race and the caliber of the competitors can be a notch below what you will encounter in your primary event.

ACTION GOALS

On a daily or weekly basis, it's important to have micro-goals that create focus for each ride or week of riding. These action goals create a common thread that ties together daily workouts and mid-term goals. They provide a daily link to your dream goals. Every workout has an objective—a specific number of intervals, a minimum mileage, and a specific heart rate or a particular skill to train and develop. The details of your daily training become your action goals.

Many athletes are very good at establishing dream goals, but they get sidetracked and never reach these goals because they have turned goal-setting into a static process. Daily evaluation should be integrated into your training program. Many factors make it necessary to change daily workouts. Planning is always an ongoing, fluid endeavor. Things change on a daily basis: races get canceled, weather affects training, or you may get sick or injured. The only way to stay on top of the variables is to change along with them.

BASIC GOAL-SETTING WORKSHEET

example

Season/Long-term Goal:

Ride a sub-40-minute 30km time trial at Nationals

Sustained concentration and effort

GOAL EVALUATION DATE: *May 2001*

What will it take to achieve my goal?
- *A solid training plan, better start technique, solid turn-around technique*
- *Improved concentration ability*

Short-term goals that will help you achieve the dream goal:
- *Research and hire a coach—start of November 2000.*
- *Have a solid training plan designed—end of November 2000.*
- *Use concentration exercises in sustained effort practices—evaluate after each practice.*
- *Find out as much as possible about Nationals' course—by February 2001.*

Is the long-term goal:

X Specific?
X Challenging, but realistic?
X Observable?
X Within your control?
X Something you're
   committed to?

Are the short-term goals:

X Specific?
X Challenging, but realistic?
X Observable?
X Within your control?
X Things you're
   committed to?

IMAGERY/VISUALIZATION

When you close your eyes, can you replay images from your last workout or race? Can you see yourself powering through the final corner of a criterium, feel the wind striking your body as you emerge from a draft, and recall the sight of the finish line approaching? Imagery is the process of recalling this stored information and reshaping it into meaningful data through a thought process. We are not talking about daydreaming about the perfect race. When used effectively, imagery is a powerful tool that involves all your senses and even your muscles.

Athletes use two types of imagery—external and internal. If using imagery means watching events unfold as if you are watching them on a home video, you are using external imagery. You are watching yourself perform an exercise from a distance. If using imagery means seeing events unfold through your own eyes, you are using internal imagery. Whichever method you use, it is critical that you include as many details as possible.

External Visualization

You can visualize a finishing sprint externally. For instance, you may see yourself battling for a wheel with half a lap to go in a criterium. Looking from overhead, you may see a hole open up on the inside of Turn Three and see yourself using that hole to move up into the top five. The peloton accelerates toward Turn Four. Riders surge to your left and you remember the thought that you need to counter them with a surge to the right. You see yourself setting up for Turn Four, careful to avoid the manhole cover in the center of the turn. You feel the force centered on your outside pedal as you fight to stay upright. You see yourself shift gears in anticipation of the uphill sprint to the finish, squeezing into a small space behind the third rider in the strung-out field. You see the overall scene of the final straightaway; remember your decision to split off to the right side of the road for your surge to the line. Just like watching a Tour de France sprint finish on television, you see yourself leap from the saddle and pound out the last 20 pedal strokes to the finish line. You see the final bike-throw and feel the exhilaration of crossing the line first. All the while you hear the roar of the crowd and the breathing of the riders near you, and you feel your heart pounding in your ears.

Internal Visualization

Now, visualize the same sprint internally. Instead of watching the last half-lap of the criterium from above, see it through your own eyes. See the rider next to you encroaching on your space, trying to move you off the wheel ahead of you. See the hole open up to your right and look through Turn Three as you accelerate into the open hole. Feel the wind hit your face as you surge to the right and counter the field's left-hand surge. Your fingers reach for the shift lever as you set up for Turn Four. Feel yourself lean into the turn and settle your weight onto your outside pedal. See the finish line come into view as you exit the turn, feel yourself rise from the saddle, and look down at your legs. See the muscles of your thighs stretch the Lycra of your shorts, see the layer of sweat and road grime coating your shins. Feel the burning in your chest and watch the other racers fading from your peripheral vision as you accelerate away from them. Focus in on the finish line ahead, and see the meters of pavement disappear under your wheels. Feel the handlebars in your hands as you push and pull against them, and feel your entire body stretching out as you throw your bike forward to cross the line first. Feel the exhilaration of winning and the relief of coasting now that the race is over.

When imagery is used effectively, it results in a physical response. You may find your heart rate increasing and feel your legs tensing as you remember each pedal stroke. Your upper body may tense in sync with your legs, as if you are pulling on the handlebars. Seeing yourself cross the finish line victorious may result in a very real sense of exhilaration, even though you are sitting on the couch.

External and internal imagery can be equally effective, and whichever you prefer to use, work on including more and more details each time you visualize. The goal is to involve all of your senses: sight, touch, smell, taste, and hearing. The more elements you can bring into the visualization, the greater the impact. Remember, mental imagery affects you physically. If you can visualize all the movements of cornering at 30 mph, you can help ingrain those patterns of movement into your muscles. Cycling takes a great deal of coordination, and imagery has been

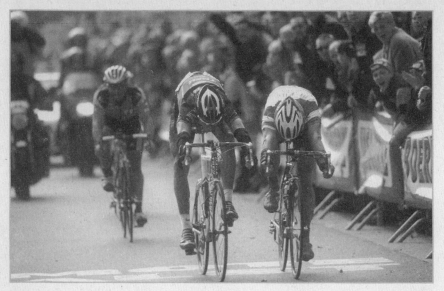

Focus on the details when using visualization; see the finish line, feel the extension of the bike throw, and hear the crowd roar. *Photo © by Graham Watson*

shown to enhance coordination, especially in sports that require complex movements.

Divers, gymnasts, and figure skaters are taught very early in their careers to use imagery. It is essential for them because their sports require extremely complex movements in rapid succession. A coaching technique I learned from a gymnastics coach is to take an athlete through a movement slowly, emphasizing exactly what has to happen, step by step. Then the athlete repeats the steps mentally, seeing how the movement unfolds slowly. The athlete's homework for the next training session is to gradually increase the speed and fluidity of the exercise in his head. During the next training session, the athlete tends to pick up the new exercise more quickly than if the coach had just had him practice it over and over again the session before. The idea is that the process of using mental imagery ingrains the sequence of movements into the brain and muscles, thereby teaching the athlete during and between training sessions to accomplish an exercise.

You're a cyclist, though, not a gymnast. No one is asking you to perform a double-twisting back somersault on a bicycle. The movements involved in cycling may seem elementary in comparison to more acrobatic sports, but refining your pedal stroke, your body position on the bike, and your tactical maneuvers can make you a more efficient and more competitive cyclist. Take your body position while climbing, for instance. Great climbers keep their upper bodies relaxed; they maintain a steady and coordinated rhythm with their legs, their breathing, and their balance on the bike. When you use imagery to practice climbing at the front of the lead group, see the movements of your feet. When are your toes pointing up, and when are they pointed down? Are you pulling through the bottom of the pedal stroke and pushing over the top? What are your hands doing? Do you have a death-grip on the bars? Are your shoulders hunched and tight, or are they relaxed? You can save a lot of energy just by training yourself to lighten your grip and relax your shoulders. It takes energy to keep those muscles contracted like that. Energy going to your shoulders is energy your legs can't use, and that is going to slow you down.

When to Use Imagery

We've already explained how you can use imagery to enhance skill development, but there are other important applications for imagery:

1. *Use Imagery During Your Warmup:* I advise all my athletes to preview as much of a racecourse as possible. For criteriums, mountain-bike races, and time trials, this often means pre-riding the course in the hours prior to competition. When you pre-ride a course, visualize what it will look like and feel like during competition. Find the manhole covers, the storm drains, the potholes, and the fastest lines through the corners. Visualize the start of the mountain-bike race as riders funnel down to the start of the singletrack. For road racers, pre-riding an entire course is unrealistic, but pre-ride at least the final five kilometers so you know the turns, where the road narrows or widens, and where you are going to be sheltered from the wind or exposed to it.

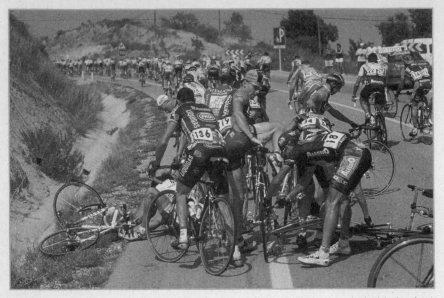

Occasional mishaps are inevitable, but being mentally prepared helps you deal with the situation quickly and calmly. *Photo © by Graham Watson*

2. *Use Imagery to Avoid Stress:* Large crowds and unfamiliar surroundings can lead to stressful situations for some athletes. If you know that there will be a huge crowd at the U.S. Track Nationals, but you usually train and race in front of sparse crowds, use imagery in your preparation. Visualize the large crowds, the noise, the banging on the boards, and the packed infield.

3. *Use Imagery to Prepare for Unexpected Problems:* I am not an advocate of practicing crashing. The truth is, most crashes happen so fast that whatever happens happens, and there isn't much you can do about it. However, what you can prepare for is how you are going to deal with the inevitable crash in competition. Visualize the crash, and then all the steps you need to take immediately afterward. Check your body for injuries, check your equipment for breakage, and make sure you have all your gear. Do you have a free lap, or do you have to chase? Is there neutral support, or do you have to supply spare wheels? Where is the pit, and how are you

supposed to get there? Now go back and replay the scenario, but change it a little. Instead of a crash, visualize the process of recovering from a flat, or of narrowly avoiding a crash and having to catch back up to the peloton. This application of imagery also works for dealing with late arrivals to race venues and other problems you may run into before, during, and after races.

When you use imagery, it is important to visualize success, but not perfection. Part of the power of imagery is that it can help prepare you for situations you have never actually experienced. Your brain doesn't really know whether stored information came from things that actually happened, things you dreamed, or things you just thought about. You may only sprint for the finish line 30 times this year, but by using imagery you can run countless scenarios of sprint finishes so you are much better prepared than a racer relying solely on the experience of 30 actual sprint finishes. And when you visualize sprinting, climbing, cornering, and battling for wheels in the peloton, you should see yourself successfully execute the maneuver. You should also, though, include errors or obstacles to success, as reality holds that you will encounter those errors and obstacles.

STRESS MANAGEMENT

Training is a process in which the proper application of stress and recovery leads to positive adaptations and improved fitness. It is important to remember that all forms of stress fit into this equation. If you are going through a highly stressful period at work, that stress has an effect on your training. I have seen a lot of athletes overload themselves because they failed to adjust their training for additional stress in their lives. I've mentioned this before, and it applies here too: training has to be integrated into your life; it cannot be approached as a separate activity that is independent of everything else you do.

The key to managing stress is to focus on the things you can control. You can't control flat tires, mechanicals, or the fact that the guy ahead of you slid out in Turn Three. You can control the factors involved in your preparation: your training schedule, nutrition, and mental preparation.

The first step to managing stress is identifying the things and situations that are stressful for you. The following is a list of the most common sources of stress for athletes, and some suggestions for dealing with the situations:

1. *Academic or Career Obligations:* Unless you are already a professional athlete, your education and/or your career need to take precedence over athletic ambitions. With those priorities established, it is easier to deal with the stress of balancing your athletic goals with classes and/or work.

   Ann Marie Miller is one CTS member who has found a way to balance her priorities and achieve her athletic goals. At 47 years old, Ann Marie trained for and won the Masters National Road Race Championship while working more than 40 hours per week at a busy New York City health club. Prioritization and great time management were the keys to her success. She made training a priority and set aside what time she could to focus on cycling. Her commitment to her goals led to her first, but probably not her last, Stars and Stripes jersey.

2. *Lack of Support (Emotional, Financial, etc.):* The people around you will not always understand the goals you have established for yourself. It is difficult to strive toward a goal that others don't find valuable. Sometimes overcoming this stressor is a matter of thoroughly explaining why your goals are so important to you and the roles the people around you play in those goals. The key to remember here is that the people around you may believe that your personal goals supersede your goals around relationships, work, or school. Part of explaining your goals is explaining where they fit in with the rest of your life goals.

3. *Family Obligations:* I am a firm believer that family always comes before anything else. Sacrificing family relationships for cycling is

shortsighted and unwise. A CTS member coached by Craig Undem wrote in a member report:

> I enjoy cycling and being fit, but my family comes first. I was concerned that my coach wouldn't understand that, and would make me feel guilty for skipping workouts. So I was surprised the first time my coach said he wanted me to skip a Saturday ride to spend more time with my daughters. I hadn't even mentioned to him that I hadn't gone to a single softball game that spring, but he said he picked it up from my comments over the previous week. Since then, we talk about my family and my job as well as my training every week, and I have been able to improve my fitness and not miss anything in this important period of my daughters' lives.

4. *Sponsor/Team Obligations:* Professional athletes are paid to perform certain roles on teams. Amateur teams like to pattern themselves after professional teams, but there is one major difference: they are not paying your bills. Keep your team's demands in perspective.

5. *Time-Management Problems:* This is where prioritization is most important. Schedule your training sessions as appointments with yourself, and stick to the schedule. Focus your training so you can accomplish as much as possible with the least amount of wasted time.

6. *Previous Performances:* Poor previous performances lead athletes to question if they have the ability to do better, and great previous performances lead athletes to worry about their ability to reach that level the next time. Write down the things you did well, and the things you need to work on following each event. Then put that performance behind you and focus on the next one.

7. *Interruptions of Habits:* You won't always get the chance to perform your perfect race warmup, or always have exactly what you want

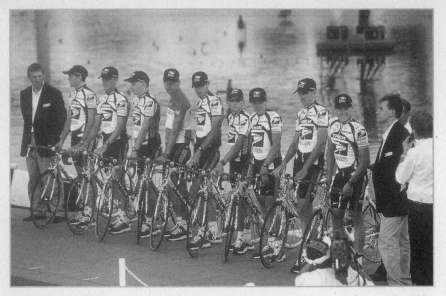

Professional cyclists are paid to work for their team leader. As an amateur cyclist, you should be careful about sacrificing your goals for those of your teammates. *Photo © by Graham Watson*

in your water bottles. Get over it. Focus on what you have going for you and the preparation you did to get where you are. Established routines are helpful, but don't be a slave to them.

8. *Interruptions of Training:* Try your best to stick to your training program, but realize that illnesses, injuries, and other obligations will sometimes interrupt your training. Avoid the urge to overcompensate for lost training time. Doubling up on mileage won't make up for a missed workout, but it may make the problem worse. Arriving at your primary event 5-percent undertrained is much better than missing the event altogether due to overtraining or an incomplete recovery from an injury.

All the aspects of mental skills training work together to help you arrive at a state of competitive readiness. When you set up your goals and expectations properly, and when you use imagery and visualization to prepare for expected and unexpected situations, you will find that you don't have a hard time with stress. If you find that you are troubled by stress, reexamine your expectations and your goals. I have often found that people become stressed when their expectations do not match the goals and situations they are mentally prepared for. If you expect to medal at the National Championships but you have not trained adequately or prepared yourself mentally for the challenge, then you are probably going to experience a lot of anxiety as the event approaches. I have also found that athletes spend too much time worrying about things they cannot control. Focus on what you can affect—your training, diet, and preparation—and understand that by doing so you will have more capacity to handle things you cannot control.

3

On the Road: Building Your Foundation of Success

KNOWLEDGE IS THE KEY to effective training, and I believe that athletes have to understand the physical effects of training in order to make the greatest gains. Gaining a working knowledge of exercise physiology and sports nutrition, as well as the components of training and periodization, is important because it gives you the ability to recognize signs of progress and/or problems. This chapter is essential to the success of your training. In later chapters, I present sample training programs for intermediate and advanced cyclists, and this chapter explains how you can adapt those programs directly to your own goals and ambitions.

Having a Ph.D. in exercise physiology won't help you become a great cyclist unless you know how to apply textbook lessons to your training. Using sports science effectively is a matter of understanding the principles and components of training, and more important, understanding the things that should and should not be manipulated in the course of developing your training program.

EXERCISE PHYSIOLOGY BASICS

Learning the basics about your body's physiology and how your body responds to daily workouts will help you better understand the CTS training methodology. In order to understand the training process, you should understand the physiology of cycling performance. What are your energy systems, and how do they work? What muscle groups power you as you ride? How do you best train them?

Aerobic Conditioning and Capacity

There are three energy systems used during cycling, ATP/CP (adenosine triphosphate and creatine phosphate), aerobic, and anaerobic. All produce adenosine triphosphate (ATP), which fuels muscle contraction. Since muscles can only store enough ATP/CP for eight to ten seconds of work, your body has to produce ATP constantly. The aerobic energy system is the primary energy-production pathway for sustained efforts. Short maximal efforts are largely dependent upon the anaerobic energy system. The ATP/CP system provides energy for only the shortest of maximum efforts. You use a combination of all three energy systems while training and competing. Unfortunately, it is difficult to train the three systems to their maximum potential simultaneously.

A poorly developed aerobic system is the primary limiting factor for success in endurance cycling. The aerobic system is responsible for the inspiration of oxygen, its absorption, its transportation, and its delivery to working muscles. When you break down all the factors of endurance performance, the more you can improve your body's ability to transport and absorb oxygen into your muscles, the better you will perform. The more work you can produce while staying in an aerobic state, the greater opportunity you have for success.

The only problem with training and developing the aerobic energy system is that it takes a long time and plenty of effort to see an increase in aerobic power output. Learning about the energy systems will help you better understand the purposes of the workouts you perform, and that will have a positive effect on your commitment to training and your ability to focus on maintaining specific training intensities. By combining knowledge of your body's energy systems, the principles of training, and periodization, you can understand how and why you apply training components like intensity, volume, frequency, terrain, and pedaling cadence in structuring your training program. Depending on your fitness and performance goals, your program needs to reflect proper training of the aerobic energy systems along with addressing the other demands of your cycling event.

The Energy Systems

ATP/CP system: For immediate energy, you use the ATP/PC system. Adenosine triphosphate and creatine phosphate fuel short, high-intensity efforts lasting ten seconds or less, such as sprinting, jumping, or short steep climbs on a mountain bike. The breakdown of the ATP molecule releases energy that the muscle can use for contraction, and the breakdown of the PC molecule releases enough energy to put the ATP molecule back together so the process can begin again. While this system is immediate, it runs out of fuel very quickly as there are only small amounts of ATP and PC stored in muscle cells. The benefits of the ATP/PC system are that it provides a lot of power for very short bursts of effort, and it gives your other anaerobic energy pathway enough time to get warmed up.

Anaerobic metabolism: After ten seconds of work, the ATP/PC system is depleted and you have to find another way to produce energy. You start breaking down stored sugar (glycogen) to produce the ATP needed for muscle contraction. Producing ATP through aerobic pathways requires more than 20 steps at the cellular level. Sometimes there just isn't enough time to wait. In the first few minutes of exercise, or during hard efforts, you may need energy faster than you can produce it utilizing oxygen. Glycolysis, another term for the anaerobic breakdown of glycogen, produces a lot of energy very quickly without utilizing oxygen. Unfortunately, this system consumes carbohydrates very rapidly, and it produces lactic acid as one of many by-products. The accumulation of lactic acid in the muscles and blood eventually limits your muscles' ability to contract, thereby forcing you to reduce your exercise intensity. This effect of the accumulation of lactic acid defines your lactate threshold (LT), and the physiological limit to how hard you can exercise for a prolonged period of time. Training can increase the amount of power you can produce, as well as the length of time you can sustain that power output. Training the anaerobic energy system with workouts near your LT improves your speed, sustainable power, and sprinting ability.

Anaerobic training is essential for all endurance cyclists, and it must be integrated into a training program that balances the aerobic and anaerobic demands of the sport. The Tour of Flanders is a very hilly World Cup race the weekend prior to the cobblestones of Paris-Roubaix. These races, with the Ghent-Wevelgem sandwiched between them, combine for one of the hardest weeks on the international racing calendar. George Hincapie thrives in the punishing environment of northern Europe in the early spring. The races are long—more than 200 kilometers—and require a huge aerobic energy output. But the unrelenting pace and incessant attacks mean repeated maximal efforts that require energy from the anaerobic system. George's aerobic training for events like the Tour of Flanders, Ghent-Wevelgem, and Paris-Roubaix is enormous, but we also integrate high-intensity interval workouts into his training to develop his anaerobic energy system. Many times, the difference between winning and finishing second is the smallest of margins. In 2001, George won Ghent-Wevelgem in a photo finish.

Aerobic metabolism: The aerobic system is the backbone of all cycling training. If your fitness goals include road racing, mountain biking, touring, or even track racing, the aerobic energy system is the primary target of your training program. After about five minutes of exercise, the aerobic system is providing the majority of the energy. It takes that long for the cardiovascular system to respond to the increase in activity and transport the oxygen to working muscles, so they can go through the 20-some steps it takes to produce ATP. The aerobic system takes longer to start producing energy, but it provides more energy per molecule of glucose than the anaerobic system does. It is much more fuel-efficient, and it produces only carbon dioxide and water as by-products—no lactic acid.

This means that the aerobic system could theoretically run forever if there were enough fuel and oxygen around. The aerobic energy system uses carbohydrate, fat, and protein to provide energy when training at low- and moderate-intensity levels. The exact percentages of fuels burned vary with availability and exercise intensity. Generally, they are most balanced when riding at low to moderate intensities, and the percentage of energy coming from carbohydrate increases as intensity goes up. Endurance training improves your efficiency for burning fat, which helps spare the glycogen stores in your muscles. This is important because the anaerobic energy system can rapidly produce energy from glycogen or glucose, but not from fat. If you have been burning fat and protein through the aerobic system, you will have some glucose left for the anaerobic system to use in the final sprint.

The CTS coaching philosophy regards the aerobic system as the cornerstone of endurance performance. No other physical aspect of cycling performance offers the returns you can reap from developing your aerobic engine. Training the aerobic energy system improves endurance, hill-climbing, time-trialing, and overall efficiency. Your body's aerobic system requires large amounts of specific training to increase its rate of oxygen delivery, absorption, and efficiency. Building a strong aerobic engine takes the right mixture of training intensity, volume, and recovery. The stronger you build your aerobic foundation, the higher you can build your Pyramid of Success.

THE ORGANIZATION OF TRAINING

Since there are physiological rules governing your performance, it makes sense that you need an organized method to improve performance within those rules. First, there are five principles that you need to abide by for your activities to be considered "training." The principles of training can then be applied to your daily activities through the manipulation of five workout components. Lastly, there's the concept of periodization: arrangement of the days, weeks, months, and years of your activities so you're applying the principles of training correctly over any given period of time.

THE FIVE PRINCIPLES OF TRAINING

When I started coaching with the U.S. Cycling Team, there was not much of an overriding structure to the team's training. I started looking at the methods used by other nations, and I realized that although each nation's program was unique, they were all united by a few core principles. When you distill the world's most successful training programs, across all sports, you arrive at five distinct principles of training:

1. Overload and recovery
2. Individuality
3. Specificity
4. Progression
5. Systematic approach

Overload and Recovery Principle

The human body is designed to respond to overload. Just take a look at bones. As you grow up, your hip and leg bones respond to your increased body weight by laying down calcium in a stronger and stronger matrix. Studies have shown that, as you grow older, continued weight-bearing exercise helps preserve that strong calcium lattice. In contrast, insufficient load has the opposite effect. Bones have been shown to be weakened by prolonged periods with no weight-bearing activity, such as a few months in space. As long as you properly overload a system in the body and allow it time to adapt, the system will grow stronger and be ready for the same or greater stress in the future.

All forms of physical training are based on your body's stress (or overload) adaptation system. To gain positive training effects, you must overload a muscle group or energy system. The overload principle applies to individual training sessions as well as to entire periods of your training. For instance, an LT interval workout needs to be hard enough and long enough to lead to adaptation. The number of intervals and interval sessions per week are also important, because it may take more than one workout session to induce enough load to lead to training adaptations.

Organizing training into blocks of similar workouts was one of the changes we made to the U.S. National Team programs in the early '90s. When I was racing, the common training program was structured to hit all aspects of cycling every week. Monday was a rest day, Tuesday was hill training, Wednesday was a long day, Thursday was for intervals, and Friday was a short ride to rest up for racing or group rides on the weekends. The limit of that program was that there was never enough load on any one energy system to lead to significant growth. A full week was too long to wait between climbing repeats for one workout to build on the benefits from the previous one. When we started restructuring training weeks to tilt the balance to specific energy systems, the athletes made significant gains very quickly.

In order to benefit from overloading an energy system, you have to give that system time to rest. When you are out on the road with the hammer down in the middle of a PowerInterval™, you are not improving your fitness. You are applying stress. Later, when you are home reading bedtime stories to your kids, you are improving your fitness. Gains are made when you allow enough time for your body to recover and adapt to the stresses you have applied. This is why I don't separate recovery from training. Recovery is part of your training, and thinking of it in those terms helps you remain as committed to recovering as you are to working out.

I once encountered an athlete who very proudly told me he had not missed a day on the bike in two years. I asked if he meant he had not skipped a training session in two years, and he clarified that he had ridden his bicycle every day of the past two years, no days off. I asked him how his racing season was going, as it was August at the time, and he rattled off a list of setbacks and illnesses that had plagued him for the past several months. He hadn't made an ounce of progress in over a year because he had never allowed his body any time to adapt to the training stress. Athletes tend to have little problem overloading systems, but they have more trouble with the recovery part.

Individuality Principle

The individuality principle seems pretty obvious, but I have always been surprised at how many athletes totally ignore it. Your buddy's training program was not designed to help you succeed, it was written for him or her. The program that will work for you has to be written and designed individually for you. Training is not a one-size-fits-all product. All parts of your program—the total hours, the number and type of intervals, and even the terrain and cadence—need to be individual. That doesn't mean that you can't train with your friends or training partners, it just means that you have to stay true to your own training program, even in their presence.

I encourage riders to find training partners so they don't have to do all of their training alone (although some training should definitely be done solo). A partner helps with motivation and the preservation of sanity. Since training partners are often on different training schedules, I suggest riding out of town together to a place you can both complete your workouts. If you are both doing flat or rolling intervals, but of different intensities and durations, do them on the same stretch of road. Pick a meeting place for after the intervals, and ride home together. Riding with a friend or group is good for you, but be careful not to let it keep you from completing the workouts that are going to make you the fastest member of that group.

Lance Armstrong's training program is designed individually for him, and when other riders try to emulate his training volume and intensity, the results are not nearly as positive. Roberto Heras learned this lesson in 2001. Roberto's climbing prowess and time trial skills put him in the elite group of racers who have the ability to win Grand Tours. He won the 2000 Tour of Spain and joined the U.S. Postal Service team as Lance's number-one lieutenant for the 2001 Tour de France and the team's leader for the 2001 Tour of Spain. Roberto and Lance spent a lot of time training together in the winter of 2000–2001; Lance followed the plan we laid out together, and Roberto followed Lance. Lance's training was wrong for Roberto; at times the load was way too high and at other times the focus was on the wrong energy systems. Roberto's 2001 season did not go as he or the Postal Service planned it. He was not on top form for the Tour de France, and the fact that he handled that race as well as he did is a testament to his talent. The Tour of Spain did not go as planned either. Roberto was the team leader, but he faltered in the third week of the race and his teammate Levi Leipheimer assumed the role of team leader. It was a great opportunity for Levi, but a disappointment for Roberto.

Roberto Heras refocused his training after the 2001 season. He still rode with training partners, but he followed a plan that met his physiological needs. He arrived at the start of the 2002 Tour de France in absolutely perfect form. He played it cool for the first ten days and then blew the race apart when the peloton hit the mountains. The Postal team lined up on the front of the peloton at the base of the final climb of Stage 11, the Tourmalet. One by one Lance's teammates pulled off, and then it was Roberto's turn. Within 500 meters, the lead group was down to just Heras, Armstrong, and the ONCE team's Joseba Beloki. Roberto set a blistering pace all the way to the finish, and he would have won the stage if the two men he was with weren't seconds apart fighting for the yellow jersey. Following the stage, Lance was not only thrilled with Roberto's performance, but he also admitted he had to tell his friend to slow down a few times. Roberto had an absolutely stellar performance in the 2002 Tour de France, largely due to the hard work he had done following an individual training program.

Specificity Principle

Your training must resemble the activity you want to perform. In a broad sense, this means that if you want to be a road cyclist, you need to spend a lot of time on two wheels. In a closer sense, it means you have to determine the exact demands of the activity you wish to perform, and tailor your training to address those demands. Be careful to examine those demands closely, because the simple answer is often too vague. For example, when you apply the principle of specificity to a cycling event like the Kilometer on the velodrome, it appears to be a simple time-trial event that lasts about one minute and three seconds. The quick and easy application of specificity would be to train for this event much like a sprinter would, focusing on anaerobic power since the race is so short and is performed at maximal efforts. But the correct application of specificity goes much deeper. The Kilo is historically won during the last 100 to 150 meters, or the last five to eight seconds of the race. Examining the energy systems used during the event, you see about 90 to 95 percent of the event uses the anaerobic system, but 5 to 10 percent

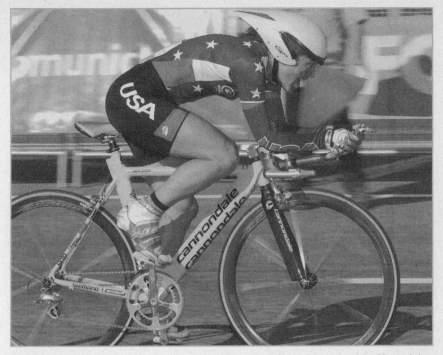

Mari Holden on her way to winning the 2000 Time Trial World Championship. Her training specifically targets the energy systems and skills necessary for success in time-trial competitions. *Photo © by Graham Watson*

of the event is primarily powered by the aerobic system. The anaerobic system can sustain only 45 to 55 seconds of work, so aerobic fitness is a factor for fast finishes. Thus, the correct application of the specificity principle is not to spend 100 percent of training time developing the anaerobic system, but instead to spend considerable time training and developing the aerobic system. The world's most successful Kilometer time trial riders are anaerobic powerhouses with highly developed aerobic systems because they train specifically for the exact demands of their discipline.

Despite training one energy system or cycling demand, specificity and variety are not mutually exclusive. Variety is a mental necessity, and I advocate varying workouts to ensure enthusiastic training. Too much of any one form of training is boring, and boredom in training will cause you to lose effectiveness in your workouts. Regardless of the training period, there are always several ways to hit the same energy system.

Progression Principle

Training needs to progressively move forward. To enjoy further training gains, you need to increase training loads as you adapt. This can mean increasing the volume of your training, or the intensity, or both. As adaptation occurs, you need to increase the number of intervals, reduce the rest between intervals, increase the length of individual intervals, or increase the intervals' intensity. Later in this chapter we will discuss the components of training and how they can be manipulated to gradually increase your training load.

The long-term application of the progression principle can be shown in the early training of a teenage George Hincapie. Early in his cycling career his endurance training was generally done with rides of two to four hours. As George progressed and matured, so did the length of his endurance rides. His endurance rides now range from two to eight hours. The duration of his Tempo (T) workouts also increased as his aerobic development progressed. Ten years ago, a 45-minute Tempo effort was adequate to overload his aerobic system. These days, we have to schedule 120-minute T efforts to produce the same training effect.

Systematic Approach Principle

When athletes start training, a haphazard training schedule produces results. Just the act of getting on the bike for a few hours each week, or throwing in a few intervals here and there, is enough to develop fitness. Pretty soon, though, that progress plateaus. Just as an architect follows a step-by-step blueprint when designing a house, your training must take a systematic approach. A successful training program must be well thought out and organized to reach your training goals. To achieve a high level of fitness, your body must advance though a planned series of training periods followed by recovery periods. If you wake up each day and simply flip a coin to determine your daily workout, you will soon find that your training progress will be limited. I have found that developing a year-round training program, based on the theory of periodization, leads to far greater progress than short-term, weekly or monthly programs. This is where having a coach becomes very valuable. Athletes need to be able to focus their attention on the short-term, daily process of training, but someone has to be looking down the road at the long-term destination of a training program. I strongly believe that one of the benefits of having a coach is having someone to entrust the long-term planning to. This allows you to focus your energy on accomplishing the short-term goals of completing your daily workouts. In the end, a systematic approach to training reduces the chance of outside variables interrupting your workouts.

THE FIVE WORKOUT COMPONENTS

When I decided to start my own coaching company, I sat down and compiled a list of specific workouts that address development of the energy systems necessary for success in endurance sports. The workouts provide a backbone for training programs, and using them effectively with athletes is a matter of manipulating variables to adjust the load applied within each workout. In order for workouts to address the principles of training, each must contain five essential components:

1. Intensity
2. Volume
3. Frequency or repetition
4. Terrain
5. Pedal cadence

You can completely change the goal of a workout by changing one of its components. For instance, climbing intervals that are ten minutes long can target two completely different energy systems if you simply change the cadence. Climbing with a cadence of 70 revolutions per minute (rpm) will tend to push an athlete to her climbing LT, which is slightly higher than her flat-ground LT due to an increase in muscle recruitment. I prescribe such workouts to develop an athlete's ability to sustain prolonged climbing efforts in races. But if the same climbing workout is done with a cadence of 50 rpm, the tension applied to the leg muscles increases greatly, and the stress on the cardiovascular system decreases. I use slow-cadence climbing efforts to increase leg strength and muscular power development. In this case, varying the cadence of an effort transforms an LT workout to an on-the-bike resistance training workout. Not only does the purpose of the workout change, but so does the training period that the workout applies to. MuscleTension™ (MT) workouts are generally prescribed in the Foundation Period, while ClimbingRepeats™ (CR) are used in the Preparation and Specialization Periods. We will cover the concept of periodization more completely later in this chapter.

Intensity

Intensity is simply a measure of how hard you are working. You can cruise down the road for 45 minutes at a comfortable spinning pace, or you can hammer along at a cross-eyed pace for 45 minutes. The energy system you are training is directly related to the intensity at which you are working, and over the years we have been able to become increasingly precise in the methods we use to measure intensity. The most widely used methods are Rate of Perceived Effort (RPE), heart rate, and power. Techniques for making use of heart rate and power will be discussed in detail in Chapter Four.

The least sophisticated method of judging intensity is RPE. You can judge RPE on various scales: 1 to 10, 1 to 16, or 6 to 20, depending on the training or testing protocol you subscribe to. While RPE provides a convenient and cost-free way to determine exercise intensity, it is difficult to use RPE to efficiently train a specific energy system. It is a subjective measure and is therefore altered by your mood and motivation.

Heart rate is more precise than RPE as a measure of training intensity. Heart rate monitors have been widely available for more than 15 years, and their use has been studied and refined a great deal. Heart rate training intensities are often determined as percentages of an athlete's maximal heart rate or LT heart rate. I have found, though, that submaximal field tests are an accurate and easily repeatable method of determining training intensity. Field tests are less invasive than maximal heart rate tests and don't require the expensive laboratory equipment necessary for accurate LT tests.

Training with power is the gold standard for determining training intensity. Powermeters measure the amount of work you are doing to propel your bicycle, and they remove several of the variables that undermine the accuracy of training with heart rate. Heart rate can be influenced by caffeine, hydration, motivation, and temperature, but power is a direct measure of the work you are actually doing, as you are doing it. Training with power provides a very accurate snapshot of an athlete's current state of fitness and fatigue, and it can be used to determine not only the recommended training intensity for a workout, but also the point when fatigue has overcome your ability to continue training effectively.

In 1999, Lance Armstrong surprised a lot of people when he won the Tour de France, but five days before the Tour began I received confirmation that he was going to win. We had set up a field test for Lance on a mountain called La Madone near Nice, France. We had used the same climb for several previous field tests, so I had a baseline of power and heart rate files to compare this test with. Lance went out, hammered his way up the mountain, rode home, and e-mailed me the data from his downloadable powermeter. Comparing that test with previous tests, it was clear that Lance was in the best shape of his life. His average heart rate was the same as it had been in earlier tests, but his power output was close to 20 watts higher than it had been just three months earlier, and it was higher than I had ever seen it. The data showed that he burned the same amount of energy as before, but that he used that energy to produce more work than ever before. It was confirmation that the training had worked, and it was a confidence boost for Lance because he knew he was going to the Tour de France with the power and fitness to win.

Volume

Training volume represents the amount of exercise done during a given workout, training week, month, or year. Some people like to think of volume in miles or kilometers, but I believe it is more useful to measure volume in hours. Twenty miles could take 40 minutes or two hours to cover depending on the terrain or weather, and as a coach I am more concerned with the amount of time you spent at a given intensity level than how far you traveled during that time.

Manipulating training volume is a way to increase or decrease your training load. If you are working on developing your aerobic engine, the intensity of your workouts has to be below your lactate threshold. Increasing the intensity causes a change in the energy system you are using. Consequently, you have to find another variable to manipulate in order to increase the load on your aerobic system. Instead of making the workout harder, make it longer. The example I used to illustrate the principle of progression applies again here. Ten years ago, a 45-minute Tempo effort was adequate to overload George Hincapie's aerobic system. These days, we have to schedule 120-minute Tempo efforts to produce the same training effect.

Volume and intensity are often inversely related. There are a lot of times when increasing volume necessitates a reduction in intensity, and sometimes you have to reduce volume when you increase intensity. If you look at an entire year of a bike racer's training, the volume tends to be highest in the Foundation and Preparation periods, when the cyclist is not racing and intensity is the lowest. When the racing season is in full swing, training volume tapers off. The intensity is so high during the height of the competition season that volume has to be reduced to prevent overtraining.

Frequency/Repetition

Frequency refers to the number of times a workout is performed in a given period of training, while repetition refers to the number of times an exercise is repeated in a single session. Three MT workouts in a week is the frequency; four MT intervals in a single workout is repetition. Both of these variables can be used to determine the method you use to manipulate the volume component of your training. More specifically, frequency and repetition are used to ensure the quality of your training sessions. During a block of MT training, you may want to accumulate three hours of MT in a week. Lumped into one workout, this is an impossible workload because you would fatigue well before you got through 30 minutes. The main purpose of using intervals is to allow for recovery time so you can repeat the same intensity level over and over again. Two sets of three 10-minute MT intervals (repetition), spaced out over three workout sessions (frequency), add up to three hours of quality MT work in a week.

Terrain

Training on varied terrain alters body position on the bike, which alters muscle recruitment. When you are climbing, you apply a lot of power to the pedals while your hands are on the tops of your handlebars. This completely changes the combination of muscles you use to support your weight on the bicycle, as well as the position of your hips and legs as you pedal. This is why two riders who can generate identical amounts of power can perform very differently on hills. If you want to excel on climbs, you have to train yourself to ride uphill well. Conversely, if you spend all your time training in the hills, you may find that you lack the ability to perform well on flat ground. A well-balanced training program includes training on varied terrain so you are prepared for racing over any kind of course.

The Tour de France covers every type of terrain found in road racing. We often refer to the first week of the Tour as "the flat stages." In reality, very few stages of the Tour are really flat; they are only flat when compared to the mountain stages. We also tend to classify racers as "climbers," "sprinters," or "rolleurs" (all-rounders). Tour riders have to be able to ride well on all terrains in order to reach the finish line in Paris. Laurent Jalabert won both the Tour de France sprinters' Green Jersey and the climbers' Polka-Dot Jersey twice in his career. He also won the three-week Tour of Spain in 1995. He exemplified the concept that the best bike racers can excel on any terrain.

Pedal Cadence

The ability to pedal at different cadences is important for your development as a cyclist. There are times when you will need the ability to muscle a large gear, and other times when it will be most beneficial to spin fast. In the beginning of this section, I used cadence to illustrate how changing one component of a workout can completely change its goal and effect. Cadence is unique in that it is not only a training variable that can help develop energy systems; it is a cycling skill in itself. Not only is it important to use cadence to develop other aspects of cycling, like your leg strength or the efficiency of your aerobic system, but it is also important to use cadence to develop an effective pedal stroke.

Lance's high-cadence climbing technique has been examined closely since he won his first Tour de France in 1999. We were motivated to develop that climbing technique as a means of shifting some of the work of climbing from his leg muscles to his cardiovascular system; the heart and lungs don't fatigue in the same manner that skeletal muscle does. It took months of specific work to change Lance's pedal stroke. He was a high-power, big-gear masher prior to cancer. After years of training, his brain, muscles, and nerves were all wired and programmed to pedal that way. Changing his pedal stroke was a matter of retraining his neuromuscular system to work in a different way. We did it by carefully focusing on the cadence component of his training. We used cadence to develop his pedaling technique as opposed to using cadence as a means to develop another energy system.

PERIODIZATION

Workout components work together to provide the elements you use every day to describe individual training sessions. The next big step to understanding the process of building a functional training program is figuring out how to arrange days and weeks of training into an organized, goal-oriented plan that addresses the five principles of training over the long term.

Periodization has been around, at varying levels of sophistication, for centuries. The scientific study of this technique began in the early 1900s and was advanced greatly by the work of Eastern Bloc scientists after World War II. Tudor Bompa emerged as the world's leading expert in periodization in 1963 while leading Eastern Bloc countries to dominating Olympic performances. His work, and the work of many other physiologists, has had enormous positive influence on training methodologies used worldwide and in almost every sport. The general concept of periodization is to break up the training year into progressively smaller segments in order to focus the training stressors. Perhaps more important, this technique organizes the scheduling of rest days and weeks to ensure that athletes get the right amount of time to adapt to their training.

Reaching your peak fitness with a periodized training plan is a matter of starting with the most general aspects of training and progressing to more specific work as you approach your goal. Seen in this manner, training for a goal event can be viewed in relation to the Pyramid of Success. Aerobic conditioning, general weight training, and basic technique work make up the base. As training progresses toward your goal event, you start moving up the pyramid. Your workouts become increasingly specific in order to overload individual energy systems. Weight training gains a speed component to produce power, and your technique work gets more advanced. As you approach your goal, everything about your training is narrowly focused on being totally prepared for the day, week, or month of your event.

In order for a periodized training program to successfully prepare you for the top of this pyramid, each level of the pyramid has to be broken down into smaller segments. I break the training year into four main periods: Foundation, Preparation, Specialization, and Transition. The Foundation and Preparation Periods work to build the endurance, strength, and power you need for competition, and your peak will come in the Specialization Period. Your training should focus heavily on one aspect of performance at a time, and after you have trained and improved that aspect, you should move on to the next aspect. The benefit of periodization is that by training the components of performance individually, you can make greater gains in each component, and subsequently you can make huge gains in overall performance.

Athletes get nervous when they focus on one aspect of training for a

YEARLY TRAINING PERIODS	TRAINING GOALS
1. Foundation	General aerobic & strength development
2. Preparation	Aerobic capacity / LT development
3. Specialization	Event-specific development
4. Transition	Active physical regeneration

Each of the four training periods of the year has specific goals associated with it.

long time. They don't like to see a month of training that includes only work on one energy system. The fear that creeps into their heads is that spending a month developing the aerobic system will ruin their ability to sprint. My point to them is, who cares if you can sprint well six months before your goal event? A stronger aerobic system and an increased capacity for riding at and above LT are both necessary components for improving your sprint. First of all, they enable you to reach the end of a race with the lead group so you have a reason to sprint. Secondly, increased power at LT correlates with increased peak power output, which means you have more power available for your final kick to the finish line. A well-structured plan includes workouts to develop your sprint only after the energy systems that support that ability have already been improved. Put another way, following a periodized training plan means developing optimal performance one energy system and skill at a time. Along the way, your capacities in individual aspects of cycling will fluctuate. But in the end, you will be stronger overall than you were before.

How Periodization Works

Within each of the four periods of training there are smaller units of time, typically four weeks apiece, each of which addresses a specific energy system or skill. These blocks of training, and each of the four weeks in any one of them, follow the theory of periodization as well. The units of a periodized training plan are often referred to in terms of cycles. Mesocycles are the largest unit; in this case, each of the four periods I refer to is a mesocycle consisting of between one and four months of training. Mesocycles are broken down into macrocycles, which are usually four weeks in length. Microcycles are the smallest unit of a periodized training plan, and they are typically seven days to correspond with a calendar week. In summary, microcycles combine to form macrocycles, and macrocycles combine to form mesocycles. And finally, mesocycles work together to form a periodized training program that leads you to success.

Weeks Every unit of a periodized plan adheres to the overload/recovery principle. Within each week of training, days are arranged to apply load and allow enough recovery time for the athlete to successfully complete all of the week's work. Depending on the athlete and time of

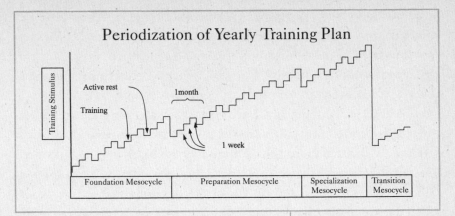

Figure 1. Typical yearly periodization scheme with micro-, macro-, and mesocycle.

year, this can mean alternating workout days and recovery days one for one, or applying training load over two or three consecutive days and then allowing one or two days for recovery.

Powermeters illustrate the benefit of consecutive days of training. For instance, I have found that athletes are capable of producing the same, if not higher, power outputs on the second day of LT training, and normally they are capable of producing that same wattage for a third day. (It is interesting to note that athletes' perceived effort increases each day during such training, but the athletes reach the same power at a lower heart rate each day of the LT training.) If I had been basing training intensity on RPE or heart rate, then actual training intensity would have been reduced on the second and third days. Using power outputs to evaluate the athletes' workouts and noticing that they were still capable of producing the same wattage each day, we continued to maintain the training intensity. After giving the athletes appropriate recovery time, I found that the consecutive days of load led to greater training adaptations. Keep in mind that the number of consecutive training days an athlete can handle varies with experience and level of development.

Months Weeks of training should be grouped together to provide a block of training that focuses on one primary energy system. These blocks are usually four weeks long; training load accumulates over the first three weeks, and the fourth week is reserved for regeneration and adaptation. During the Preparation Period, I use Tempo workouts to increase the power an athlete can produce at aerobic intensities. The key to making significant gains with T is to spend a huge amount of time riding at that workout intensity. For experienced cyclists, this can mean three T workouts a week during a three-week training block. Since T work is defined by riding at a specific intensity and cadence, increasing the length of workouts is the best way to increase training load. The first week of a T-focused Preparation Period training block may include three 30-minute sessions (Tuesday, Thursday, and Saturday, to allow for adequate recovery). In the second week, the duration of the T workouts may increase to 40 minutes each, and they may get even longer in the third week. Athletes are typically pretty tired by the end of a three-week training block, and that's why the fourth week is for regeneration.

Regeneration weeks are critical to the success of your training program. The three weeks of focused training are meant to put intense pressure on your energy systems, and it is that pressure that your body responds to during your regeneration week. A regeneration week gives you the opportunity to use the majority of your energy for growth and adaptation, instead of using every ounce of available energy to recover from one workout to the next. Therefore, it is important to give your body the ingredients it needs for growth: food, water, and rest. Don't make the mistake of reducing your caloric intake during regeneration weeks because your training hours are reduced. Regeneration weeks are not the time to skimp on food or rest.

In 2000, I was working with Ron Williams, a U.S. Paralympic cyclist who was super-motivated to have the ride of his life in the Sydney Paralympics. He moved to Colorado Springs to train at altitude and use the velodrome we have here. I gave him a few easy weeks to acclimate to the altitude and then we started applying the pressure. After a few months of hard training, it was time for one last block of training before the Paralympics. For three weeks I threw everything but the kitchen sink at this guy. He was training for the pursuit event on the track, and I was there to call out intermediate ("split") times during his velodrome workouts. During the final block of training, his split times went from medal-pace to barely fast enough to qualify, and he started to suffer. His anxiety level went up, his motivation went down, he started giving up in the middle of intervals, and he was worried that he wouldn't be able to perform in the Paralympics. Physically he was handling the training just the way I hoped he would, but he was suffering mentally because it was the first time he had ever had to work that hard. After three strenuous weeks, he moved into a planned regeneration week. By the end of that week his mood, motivation, and confidence had completely rebounded, and his split times started coming down again. A few weeks later in Syd-

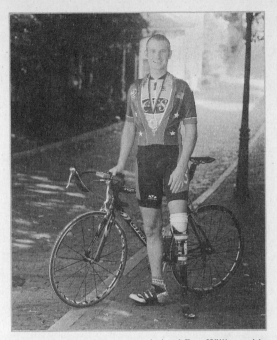

A periodized training program helped Ron Williams ride his personal best at the 2000 Paralympics in Sydney, Australia. *Photo © by Randy Crow*

ney, he rode a personal best in the 3,000-meter pursuit. Regeneration periods are the key to making huge gains, and having a good periodization plan means that those regeneration periods are scheduled to ensure that you are at your best exactly when you need to be.

Years Training needs to be arranged so that the training goal of one block builds on the fitness and development from the previous one. Achieving peak fitness is like building a skyscraper. The height of the building depends on the size and stability of its foundation and the strength of its walls. You have to start from the bottom and work your way up. In this case, I start with aerobic conditioning in the Foundation Period because I know that the LT work scheduled for the Preparation Period depends on a strong aerobic engine for success. The stronger you build the aerobic engine during the Foundation Period, the higher power output you will be able to generate through LT work. For successful VO_2 (maximum amount of oxygen consumed during exercise) work in the Specialization Period, you are still depending on the supporting structure of the aerobic system, as well as on your ability to produce high power at lactate threshold, to extend your ability to sustain, repeat, and recover from maximal efforts. The height of your peak depends on the strength of your program, and your program derives its strength from your periodization plan.

Each period of the training year has a broad training goal, and each month in the period is focused on training that contributes to that goal. All CTS workouts correspond to a specific training period and they are designed to prepare you for the demands of the next training period. However, some workouts are used throughout the year to provide variety and maintain the principle of individuality of training.

ABOUT THE PERIODS

Foundation Period

The Foundation Period of your training year has the largest effect on the height of your peak. This is the period of the year that focuses on building the superior aerobic engine that will power the rest of your energy systems. Your training volume is high during this period, but the intensity of your workouts should be relatively low. I like to set heart rate ceilings for athletes I work with. A heart rate ceiling allows an athlete to ride normally, without worrying about heart rate falling on descents or at stoplights. The point of the ceiling is to keep an athlete from riding too near his LT and accumulating lactic acid. The Foundation Period is also the time of year when you should focus on strength training and pedaling mechanics. Workouts incorporated in the Foundation Period include PowerStarts™ (PS), Stomps™ (S), FixedGear™ (FG), FoundationMiles™ (FM), FastPedal™ (FP), and MT™, as well as weekend group/club rides.

I believe that long endurance miles and resistance training don't work well together. One must come before the other. Accordingly, training intensity and/or volume should be reduced as the intensity and volume of strength training increase. I recommend unique workouts, such as FP and FG, to help maintain aerobic conditioning during the heavy resistance training. At CTS, our coaches also incorporate unique "on-the-bike" resistance training into programs. You gain the strength benefits from weight training and have the added advantage of functional strength training on your bike! This means you are not only stronger in the weight room, but that your strength transfers directly into the pedals.

The French track cycling team has combined strength training and cycling in a unique and effective way. They set up weight training equipment in the infields of their velodromes, and the athletes go directly from lifting weights to on-the-bike power work on the track. As a result, French track cyclists are among the most powerful in the world. You can use a similar technique in your Foundation Period training by performing your weight training on the same days that you do S, PS, or MT workouts. When athletes lift weights before going out and doing on-the-bike resistance workouts, their power outputs on the bike are higher than when they perform only the cycling workouts. The effectiveness of the cycling workouts increases because of neuromuscular adaptation; the weight training improves your central nervous system's ability to recruit muscle fibers.

Since the intensity of your cycling workouts is relatively low during the Foundation Period, it is a great time of year to focus on pedal mechanics. FP workouts improve the efficiency of your pedal stroke and stress your aerobic system without putting tension on your leg muscles. The high cadence stresses your cardiovascular system, but since you are breaking up the work of pedaling into small pieces, the stress on your leg muscles is reduced. OneLeggedPedaling (OL)™ drills work each leg independently to isolate weaknesses in specific portions of your pedal stroke. Regeneration weeks are good times to incorporate pedaling drills. Since the duration and intensity of your workouts decrease, you should focus on the form and efficiency of your pedal stroke during these periods of active recovery.

Studies at the Olympic Training Center have shown that you don't produce positive work throughout the entire pedal stroke. Pulling up during the upstroke doesn't add any positive force because the downstroke is so powerful that you are actually lifting the opposing leg. The best you can do is partially unweight the leg being lifted. The portions of the pedal stroke where you can increase your power output are through the top and bottom. OneLeggedPedaling (OL) workouts help you focus on improving these two areas of the pedal stroke.

Lance Armstrong's aerobic conditioning rides during the Foundation Period incorporate pedaling drills like FP and OL, and I restrict his gearing so his cadence remains high for hours at a time. I also instruct him to stay seated at all times, even on short hills where he is tempted to stand up and power over the top. He even installs a cassette with a 25-tooth cog on it so he can stay seated and maintain a high cadence on hills while remaining aerobic.

Although the aerobic system is the primary training target during the Foundation Period, the energy systems are not 100-percent independent of one another. The aerobic and anaerobic energy systems influence one another, and it is important to periodically add training workouts that stress all energy systems, regardless of your current training period. It is typically best to train this area using weekend club rides or training races because these activities include various changes in speed and power. Group rides are a fun break from regimented training throughout the year, and they provide opportunities to utilize all of your energy systems.

The length of your Foundation Period depends on your overall fitness and experience level. Generally, 16 weeks of Foundation training is sufficient to build the aerobic engine and base of strength to support more intense work in the Preparation Period. Four months allows enough time to complete blocks of endurance, on-the-bike resistance, pedal mechanics, and Tempo training.

Preparation Period

During the Preparation Period, the focus of your training starts to narrow as you prepare for competition. The intensity and volume of training increase, and the workouts begin to include demands that are similar to what you will experience in competition. The amount and quality of the aerobic development work that you did during the Foundation Period weighs heavily on the success of your Preparation Period. You may find yourself overly tired in a few weeks, and possibly overtrained in a few months, if you're not ready for the increased intensity and volume of the Preparation Period.

How can you tell if you've done enough work in the Foundation Period and are ready to move on? Many times it's a matter of planning. Spending 16 weeks building your aerobic engine should be sufficient, and then you should be ready to move on to the Preparation Period. One way to prove you are prepared is to look at training data from the Foundation Period. You should see that your sustainable power, during aerobic efforts like Tempo workouts, has increased consistently. When your power stops increasing consistently, it is time to move on to the Preparation Period. You have already reaped great results from your aerobic training, and any more work would cost you more in workout time and energy than you would gain in power output.

Since you have built a huge and powerful aerobic engine, the Preparation Period is the time to put it to good use. Sustainable power at lactate threshold is the goal of this period, and as a result, your training must include frequent and long intervals near your threshold intensity. Due to the increased intensity, as compared with the Foundation Period, adequate recovery becomes increasingly important during this time of year. LT workouts can be done on consecutive days, sometimes up to three days in a row, but you have to increase the amount of recovery time between blocks of consecutive training days.

Beyond recovery, there are two main issues that hinder many athletes' LT workouts during this critical time of year: intensity and duration. To be effective, these workouts have to be done at an intensity that can be maintained for a long period of time. It is the amount of time at that intensity, and not the intensity itself, that leads to gains in power at lactate threshold.

The problem with LT training is the lactic acid itself. As soon as the intensity rises above LT, the concentration of lactic acid in muscle cells negatively affects the muscles' ability to contract. You lose the ability to continue exercising at that intensity, and either the workout must be cut short or the intensity must be reduced. Accumulating a lot of lactic acid also increases the recovery time necessary before you can effectively train again. This means that training your LT power has to be done at intensities below your actual lactate threshold.

Training can alter your LT heart rate, but only a little bit. Training's greater effect is to increase the amount of work you can do, and the amount of time you can sustain that work, at your LT heart rate.

SteadyState™ (SS) and ClimbingRepeat™ (CR) workouts develop your power at lactate threshold because they teach your body to operate at its maximum sustainable effort level for long periods of time. You are training on a relatively thin edge. If you back the intensity down a notch, your aerobic engine could sustain the effort for hours. If you increase the intensity a few heart beats or watts, your muscles would fill with lactic acid within minutes. But when the intensity is just right, you're creating a lot of lactic acid and your body is increasing its efficiency for dealing with it. What's happening is your body is converting accumulated lactate in the blood to carbon dioxide and water through several steps. Your body's reaction to increased blood concentration of carbon dioxide is to increase your breathing rate. This allows your lungs to remove the excess carbon dioxide from your blood so you can exhale it. You're learning to clear and buffer lactic acid, and you're becoming increasingly efficient at burning fuel. As a result, the amount of time you can spend working at your LT increases. More important, the amount of work you can do before you reach the threshold also increases.

To illustrate the importance of a strong aerobic system and effective LT training, take the case of a time trial rider. Let's say your goal is to win the USA Cycling Masters National Time Trial Championship, and you estimate you need to produce 325 watts for nearly an hour in order to reach your goal. You develop your aerobic engine in the Foundation Period, and by the beginning of the Preparation Period you can sustain 220 watts for 60 minutes at Tempo intensity. After eight weeks of LT work, including SS, CR, and practice time trials, you can produce 315 watts before you cross LT. You can maintain that intensity for over an hour, but when you increase your power output to 325 watts, you can stay there for only 30 minutes because you have to ride above LT to reach 325 watts.

Now let's go back through the same scenario where you can sustain 250 watts for 60 minutes at Tempo intensity, instead of 220 watts. The stronger aerobic system means you can produce more power before having to tap into the anaerobic energy system, thereby delaying the onset of lactic acid accumulation. The aerobic system is producing more work than before, so when you add the additional power that you can produce as you approach LT, the sum is greater than when you started with a weaker aerobic system. Now you can sustain 320 watts for over an hour, and because of the increased power that you can produce before crossing LT, you can sustain 325 watts for the 50-some minutes that you need to win the USA Cycling Masters National Time Trial Championship.

A goal event like that Time Trial Championship would come during the Specialization Period, but you should start entering competitions a few weeks into your Preparation Period. You are not at optimal race-fitness during this period, and the first few competitions you enter during the Preparation Period are for training and not necessarily for results. You may not have the fitness to be very competitive in those races, since your training load is high, but don't let struggling through some early-season races bother you. If you are following a periodized training plan, you are not going to race well during some portions of the year. On the other hand, there will be at least one portion of the year in which you can race better than you ever have before.

Racing always demands more from you than you can demand of yourself in training. The repeated and unexpected changes in pace, as well as the arousal of competition, are necessary to prepare you for complete readiness once your race-fitness improves. Just as your power and aerobic capacity increase as you progress toward your goal event, your racing ability will also improve through training. Competitors learn from competition, and you have to race in order to learn how to win. Enter races and take risks; this is the time of the season when you can afford to make some mistakes. Get into long breakaways, attack in the final kilometer, lead out the sprint, and try tactics you aren't comfortable with. Notice how the rest of the field responds to your actions and remember what works and what doesn't so you can use that information for your benefit in your goal event.

Your racing success depends on your knowledge as well as on the strength of your energy systems, and it is important to continually develop both. Workouts included in the Preparation Period training include: T, SS, CR, and PowerIntervals (PI)™.

Specialization Period

The Specialization Period is many people's favorite time of year. This is the period when you are able to perform at your best and when the months of regimented training pay off. Your goal event should be in the Specialization Period, and the focus of your training is on race-specific elements of fitness and optimizing your high-end energy systems. Training intensity is at its highest and the weekly training volume is reduced to accommodate the demands of increased training intensity. Your workouts should emphasize speed and repeatability—that is, the ability to repeat high-speed efforts with little recovery between efforts. This speed training is necessary because aerobic and LT training often provides little improvement for speed and racing agility. You need the ability to move quickly and confidently on your bicycle at high speeds and pedal cadences. Repeatability training is needed because races are often won or lost by your ability to initiate or respond to accelerations at critical times. The best time to attack is right after a previous attack was chased down, but that means you have to be able to hit the throttle with little or no recovery from that previous effort.

Workouts during the Specialization Period alternate between full-throttle and active recovery. These are at completely opposite extremes of the spectrum. The intensity of your full-throttle workouts has to be above race-pace, and that means your recovery rides and activities need to be easy spinning. One consequence of exercising at such extremes is that your aerobic conditioning, which is developed by intensities somewhere in the middle, begins to suffer.

The Specialization Period is the most difficult balancing act of the whole year. You have to watch very carefully for signs of fatigue and illness due to an imbalance between overload and recovery. The workouts are very intense but very short, and you may feel deceptively strong. A lot of athletes react to feeling strong by riding harder. You can't blame them; they have been training hard for months and now have the ability to ride fast, so they want to ride as fast as they can. Unfortunately, that viewpoint is shortsighted because they are increasing the training load and not increasing recovery time. It doesn't take long for that strength and power to evaporate, and instead of being ready for your goal event, you'll find that your best performances were during training races three weeks earlier.

An athlete can only hold on to an extremely high level of aerobic and anaerobic fitness for a short time. If you hit that top level of fitness too early, you won't be able to hold on to it long enough to reach your goal event in top condition. Likewise, if you are not ready to enter the Specialization Period until two weeks before your goal event, you won't have enough time to fully develop all aspects of your performance. The intensity of the Specialization Period leaves little time for workouts to maintain your aerobic conditioning, and it's very difficult to maintain deep aerobic fitness when your workouts vary between high-speed training and recovery spinning. Consequently, it is often necessary to incorporate several microcycles of long endurance training to give your aerobic system a boost during the Specialization Period. This is especially true for athletes who aim to be in great form for periods longer than four to six weeks.

Lance Armstrong needs to be in absolutely top shape for three weeks in July. In the beginning of his career, that would have been difficult because he couldn't hold on to that kind of fitness, mental fortitude, and focus for that long. Through years of training, and partially as a result of maturing as a man and an athlete, Lance has about a seven-week window for peak fitness. That is, he can pull together all the elements of optimal performance and hold on to them for about seven weeks. For that period of time, he is physically at his best and he can maintain his focus on nutrition, training, racing, tactics, travel, and the media. Toward the end of this period, his focus and motivation begin to slip because the strain of the past several weeks have worn him out. Understandably, I plan his entire year around making sure the Tour de France falls right in the middle of those seven crucial weeks.

Given the choice, I would rather Lance reach peak fitness too early as opposed to too late. If he is at risk of peaking too early, we can back off his training a little bit and delay his peak. But if his preparation falls behind schedule, there is nothing anyone can do to make up for lost time. As I've mentioned, Lance and I talk almost daily throughout the year, and during May and June we adjust his training daily to fine-tune his preparedness for the Tour de France.

Transition Period

A few weeks after the end of the Tour de France, Lance enters the Transition Period of his periodization plan. Following a period of peak fitness and hard racing, athletes need time to recuperate and refocus on the basics of training. In Lance's case, he peaks once during the year, for a relatively short period of time. Many other athletes plan for two peaks during the year, and they often return to the Preparation Period for a month or two between heavy competition periods. Still others aim for a slightly lower peak, but try to hold on to a high level of fitness for a longer period of time. This is most often the case for regional- and national-level amateur racers. Regardless of the length or intensity of your competitive season, I recommend that everyone follow it immediately with a Transition Period.

Training volume and intensity both reduce drastically during the Transition Period, since the goal of this time is to recuperate and prepare for the long buildup to your next peak. More important, your training should be unstructured and include activities outside of cycling during these four to six weeks. You don't want to detrain much during this period. You will lose your race-specific capacities after a few weeks, but even with reduced training volume you will retain a large portion of your aerobic strength. Training in the Transition Period is important because it prevents you from having to spend weeks of the Foundation Period regaining fitness that you lost unneccessarily.

Cross-training helps to build and maintain muscles that are rarely used in cycling. There is very little lateral movement on a bicycle, and as a result, cyclists tend to develop muscle imbalances. We are very powerful in one plane of movement (moving the legs perpendicular to the torso), but very weak in others (moving the legs parallel to the torso). A simple game of basketball or touch football should not leave you immobile for two days, and yet some of the most highly trained aerobic athletes I have ever known couldn't run a single mile without hurting themselves.

The Transition Period is most important for junior cyclists who are still growing. For them, the Transition Period should be two to three months long so they can participate in school sports. I encourage junior cyclists to take extensive amounts of time to participate in other sports throughout the year. I don't believe it is wise for young athletes to specialize in one sport too early. Sports are critical for the development of a child's social skills, balance, and hand-eye coordination. It is through sports, both team and individual, that children gain the balanced strength and coordination that are critical for healthy development. While I think cycling offers tremendous benefits to young athletes, I also recognize that these athletes are better served, overall, by participating in a variety of activities. There is plenty of time for young men and women to focus on cycling, but I believe it is more important for them to be athletes first, and to be experienced and competent in a variety of sports, before they focus solely on cycling.

THERE IS NO OFF-SEASON

This point deserves its own section: the "off-season" is a myth. And I am not talking about taking a vacation from training for a few weeks. A few weeks off your bike is not an off-season, it is a short break, and it is good for you. For years, people have been referring to the fall and winter as the off-season, and it doesn't make any sense. The success of your entire periodization plan depends on the size and strength of your aerobic engine, your foundation, which for most people must be built in the fall and winter.

In a December 2001 interview, Lance Armstrong said, "The point is, there is no real off-season for me. I don't think I've missed three consecutive days off the bike since the Tour de France." In the month following the Tour, Lance was on his bike almost every day, but I wasn't prescribing structured workouts for him to do. It's important for athletes to get away from the regimen and pressure of a training schedule sometimes, and unstructured training is far better than sitting on the couch for a month.

A highly trained aerobic athlete can get away with doing absolutely nothing for nine to 12 days before there will be an appreciable loss in fitness. However, it can take between eight and 12 weeks to regain fitness lost after taking four weeks off. That means if you don't exercise for the month of October, sometime in January you could be as fit as you were at the end of September. It is difficult to make significant strength and power gains from year to year if you spend three months losing and regaining fitness.

4

Tools of Training

UNDERSTANDING THE COMPONENTS and principles of training and periodization is an essential part of developing into the 100% Ready Athlete, but you have to delve into the details as you begin the process of training. First you have to establish a starting point for your fitness so you can determine the type, intensity, and frequency of training that you need to reach your goals. The coaches at CTS and I use performance testing and subsequent data interpretation to establish baseline fitness information for athletes. Once we know your initial fitness level, we can choose an appropriate method for prescribing workout intensity and select the most effective workouts and exercise conditions. It is also important to assess the roles of resistance training, flexibility, and recovery in the process of achieving your goals. Establishing your periodization plan is essential for building your Pyramid of Success, and the next step is assembling the right tools to reach the peak.

PERFORMANCE/FITNESS TESTING

There are three primary reasons for performance testing:

1. *Determining an athlete's baseline fitness level.* This helps establish initial levels of intensity and volume for your training. One of the most common mistakes that self-coached athletes make is prescribing training for themselves that is ultimately too demanding. It is rare that new CTS members come to us with training that is too easy. The majority of the time, we have to reduce significantly new members' total training load.
2. *Determining changes in fitness level, as compared to previous tests.* This allows both athlete and coach to evaluate the overall effectiveness of the training program.
3. *Determining an athlete's specific weaknesses.* One of the fundamental ideas I adhere to with all my athletes is to "train the weaknesses and race the strengths." Ideally, by making weaknesses (physiological, technical, or otherwise) a training priority, they can eventually become strengths.

Performance testing can be separated into two broad categories: laboratory testing and field testing. Laboratory testing provides wonderful information because you can directly measure an athlete's physical reaction to exercise. You can determine VO_2 max by analyzing the relative concentrations of oxygen and carbon dioxide in inspired and expired air. You can get an accurate determination of your lactate threshold by analyzing blood samples taken at increasing intensity levels. Unfortunately, laboratory tests are usually expensive, not readily available, and difficult for most athletes to incorporate into daily training. Also, the data from laboratory testing must be correlated with other measures, most commonly heart rate or power, because devices to directly measure these physiological parameters aren't readily available for use while actually training.

Field testing has several advantages over laboratory testing:

- No direct cost associated with field tests.
- Results are accurate and provide real-world data that you can easily apply to your training.
- The test can be easily repeated several times each year.
- Field tests are less invasive than laboratory testing, and less disruptive to training.

Lance Armstrong has access to the most sophisticated laboratory equipment in the world, and yet I still primarily rely on field tests to evaluate his training progress. Lance doesn't compete in a lab, and I need to know how his training is affecting his ability to ride a standard bicycle, on regular roads, in normal conditions.

THE CTS FIELD TEST

The CTS Field Test consists of two short time trials, preferably over the same course. This can be the complete workout for most cyclists, especially when you include warmup, recovery between efforts, and then a cooldown. Depending on your circumstances (weather or terrain), these can be time-based efforts (eight minutes in duration) or distance-based (three miles). I recommend a field test every six to eight weeks throughout the year.

When performing the CTS Field Test, collect the following data:

- Time of each effort (mm:ss)
- Average heart rate for each effort
- Average power (if available) for each effort
- Average cadence for each effort
- Weather conditions (warm vs. cold, windy vs. calm, etc.)
- Course conditions (indoors vs. outdoors, flat or hilly, point-to-point vs. out-and-back, etc.)
- Rate of Perceived Exertion (RPE) (how hard you felt you were working) for each effort.

You are going to repeat this field test several times throughout the year, and the data you gather needs to be comparable between tests. Repeated field tests establish baseline data that you can use to evaluate training progress. The more consistent you keep your field test location and conditions, the more accurately you can judge your progress over time. Try to reduce the number of variables between tests by using the same course under similar conditions (temperature, wind) every time. The following are instructions for the CTS Field Test:

STEP #1: Find/Create a Test Course

Locate and measure, to the best of your ability, a flat, three-mile course. Ideally, try to select roads that aren't busy and that don't involve turns. If turns cannot be avoided, then include only right-hand turns, and remember to adhere to traffic laws.

STEP #2: Perform the Test When Rested

You want to perform your test when you are relatively well rested. The end of a regeneration week is a good time for a field test, because not only are you well rested, you can also plan similar training/recovery for the days prior to field tests throughout the year. Remember, reproducibility is a key consideration, especially when you begin accumulating data from numerous field tests over time.

STEP #3: Fuel Your Body Properly

If possible, don't eat any solid foods for the two hours immediately prior to the test. However, in the 45 minutes or so immediately prior to Effort #1, consume a high-carbohydrate sports drink that you are comfortable with. Make sure you record your food intake prior to the field test, so you can duplicate this for future tests.

STEP #4: Warmup

The purpose of the warmup is to prepare yourself both mentally and physically for the challenge of the efforts to come. You want to activate your energy systems, but not cause undue fatigue. The warmup should last ten minutes at a minimum, and should include two or three high-intensity efforts. These should be one to two minutes in length, with at least two to four minutes of recovery between each two efforts (recovery time between efforts should be twice as long as each effort). Also, each effort should be performed at a relatively high cadence, or at least a cadence that is 10 to 15 rpm higher than you anticipate performing the time-trial efforts. By the end of the warmup, you should be physically warm, sweating, and prepared for Effort #1. You want around five minutes between the completion of the warmup and the start of Effort #1.

STEP #5: Begin Effort #1

From a standing start (preferably with a friend to hold you), begin with your dominant leg's crank arm at the two o'clock position so you can take advantage of your body weight on the first power stroke. Your gear selection should allow a fast, stable start—not so small that you spin the gear out before you are able to sit down, and not so large that you can barely get it moving. As you gain speed, gradually move to a sitting position as you reach your top pedal cadence for the starting gear. Once you are seated, shift into a higher gear. It's important to remember to avoid the urge to start too fast. If you reach top speed in less than 45 seconds, you started too quickly.

STEP #6: Find Your Ideal Gear

Once you are up to speed, your gearing should allow you to maintain a cadence between 90 and 95 rpm on flat terrain or between 80 and 85 rpm if climbing. Avoid the impulse to "mash," or push a big gear at low rpm. This leads to premature fatigue, which ultimately means a slower time. Over time, you will find a cadence that is most efficient for your individual style and level of ability. I suggest that for the first few tests you experiment in the range of 80 to 95 rpm, allowing a five-rpm range per effort. The most efficient rpm range for you usually means a faster time and lower average heart rate throughout the effort.

STEP #7: Achieve Maximum Sustainable Intensity

When you reach a speed that you feel you can barely maintain for the entire time of the effort, settle into a steady breathing rhythm. Most athletes subconsciously settle into their most efficient breathing rhythm and depth, so I don't recommend spending a whole lot of time concentrating on your breathing technique. From this point forward, the effort is going to be challenging. If it isn't taking a great deal of effort to maintain your speed, odds are you're not at your maximum sustainable speed. Force the pace all the way to the end of the effort.

STEP #8: Collect the Data

Complete the effort, and immediately collect the data listed above. Record the time of the effort to the nearest second. It is also good to record subjective observations that may prove insightful, including your RPE, how hard you started, and how comfortable you felt with the cadence.

STEP #9: Recover Between Efforts

Allow ten minutes of active recovery between Effort #1 and Effort #2. During this time, ride slowly and at low intensity, but keep your cadence a little higher than the rpm you selected for Effort #1. If you need to stop, keep this time to a minimum. Active recovery leads to quicker recovery than complete rest. Staying on the bike with your legs moving helps remove lactic acid from your muscles and keeps them warm for Effort #2.

STEP #10: Begin Effort #2; Collect Data

Repeat steps #4 through #7.

STEP #11: Cooldown

Once you complete Effort #2, the field test is over. Instead of ten minutes of active recovery, conclude the ride with at least 15 minutes of active recovery. Once you return home, record any additional data, such as course and weather conditions. Good job!

Moving the CTS Field Test Indoors

Sometimes it's not possible to perform a field test outdoors due to inclement weather, lack of suitable/safe course, or lack of daylight or time. When performing the field test indoors, I recommend still performing the efforts based on distance. For most stationary trainers, you will need a rear-wheel mount for your cycling computer so that you can still measure distance. If this isn't possible, then you can perform time-based efforts (two eight-minute efforts) instead. Although you won't be able to use "time" of efforts to determine improvement, you can still at least observe any changes to your average heart rate for each effort. If you have a powermeter, then you can still determine if your average watts improved.

Also, take care when adjusting your rear-wheel resistance to the load unit of the stationary trainer. If the manufacturer hasn't provided a reproducible protocol, inflate your tires to a specific pressure and then count how many turns (if applicable) you need to get firm resistance between the load unit and the tire. Record both settings so you can reproduce them for your next test. If your load unit is spring-loaded, there isn't much you can do. One last recommendation is to avoid performing your field test on rollers, unless they have an additional resistance unit attached.

HOW TO TRAIN WITH HEART RATE

Now that you've completed your field test, it's time to use the heart rate data to determine the intensity of your training. I have found over the years that using average heart rates, as opposed to maximum (or peak) heart rates, yields better responses from athletes at all ability levels and minimizes any risk of overtraining. I also prefer using average heart rates because they are indicative of an athlete's true response to the entire duration of the effort. Maximum heart rate, on the other hand, might only provide information about a few seconds of the effort. When you think about it, an effort that lasts close to eight minutes should give me more useful data than only a second or two. Maximum heart rate doesn't provide enough data to create an entire range of intensities for training.

When I was working on Lance's comeback to cycling, I wanted to increase the precision of heart rate training. Lance could handle only a limited workload, and I wanted to make sure he was using his time effectively. One of my major departures from conventional training methodology was to move away from using widely accepted "heart-rate zones." Instead, I began using "ranges" that are much narrower (3 to 6 beats) as opposed to "zones" that I found to be excessively wide (20 beats) for critical workouts. A complete list of workouts is located on pages 94–113.

For example, using the zone system based on maximum heart rate, if an athlete's peak or max HR observed during a field test was 195 beats per minute, and his target training zone is 75 to 85 percent of max HR, then this creates a training zone between 146 and 166 beats per minute . . . a 20-beat difference. My experience is that for most individuals, even if the max HR is valid and reliable for ultimately determining intensities, this "zone" is still much too wide. With a zone this wide, the relative contributions from various energy systems change considerably from one end of the zone to the other. If your goal is to develop aerobic endurance, exercising at the low end of the zone may be too easy, and exercising at the high end of the zone may be too hard.

Determining HR Ranges

To determine your various heart rate ranges and ceilings, apply the percentages listed below to the highest average heart rate from your field test. This provides the low number of the range. Next, add two to four beats to determine the high number of the range.

For example, take a senior whose average heart rates during the field test were 183 (Effort #1) and 185 (Effort #2). The lower limit of her Tempo heart rate range would be: $185 \times 0.88 = 163$ beats per minute (bpm). To generate the heart-rate range for Tempo workouts, add 2 to 4 bpm to 163 (we will add four). The Tempo heart rate range for this senior athlete becomes 163 to 167.

	SENIOR (< 35 YEARS)	MASTER (> 35 YEARS)
FoundationMiles™	≤ 89%	≤ 86%
EnduranceMiles™	≤ 91%	≤ 88%
Tempo™	88% (low) + 2–4 beats (high)	87% (low) + 2–4 beats (high)
SteadyState™	92% (low) + 2–4 beats (high)	90% (low) + 2–4 beats (high)
ClimbingRepeats™	95% (low) + 2–4 beats (high)	92% (low) + 2–4 beats (high)

I recommend using "heart rate ceilings" during FM and EM rides instead of prescribing lower limits to heart rate. These heart rate ceilings are useful because they provide a specific marker that you should stay under in order to facilitate development of the aerobic energy system. By only providing a ceiling, you have a great deal of freedom, and it is usually in the context of group rides that a ceiling is most appropriate, especially in the Foundation and Preparation Periods of training.

Your goal should be to spend at least 95 percent of the FM and EM training time below your heart rate ceiling. For example, if the total ride time is two hours (120 minutes), then you should spend at least 114 minutes below the ceiling. It's okay to have the HR go above the ceiling, especially if dictated by terrain, such as short steep climbs, etc., as long as these efforts are short (ideally less than 30 seconds) and there aren't too many of them. If you ignore the HR ceiling often, you will hinder the development of your aerobic energy system during the Foundation and Preparation Periods, and this will decrease your performance potential later in the season.

Factors Affecting Heart Rate

Many factors affect heart rate and its ability to be used as an indicator of training intensity. This doesn't mean we can't use heart rate, but it does mean we need to use caution when interpreting heart rate data from training and/or racing.

There is often a delay or "lag" between the actual change in exercise intensity and the subsequent change in heart rate (up or down), because HR response is actually a "result" of training intensity, not a determinant of the intensity itself. This means that using HR for prescribing intensity is not usually appropriate for shorter efforts (less than two minutes). This is why many of the anaerobic workouts listed later in this chapter don't have corresponding HR ranges.

Effective training impacts heart rate, both at rest and during exercise. As the cardiovascular system becomes more efficient, your resting HR decreases, and your average HR for any given workload also decreases.

Adding too much intensity and/or volume to your training program, or taking too little recovery between high-intensity workouts, causes premature fatigue and overreaching. Continuing this for more than a few weeks can ultimately lead to overtraining. Fatigue and overreaching can cause resting HR to increase and average HR for given workloads to increase.

Both resting and exercise HR can be affected by illness or medication. Many times, regardless of the effect of the medication or the metabolic implications of any disease or illness, you will notice a discrepancy between heart rate and perceived effort. For any given workload, your perceived effort will likely be higher as compared to when you are healthy. I recommend that you check with your physician if you are on any type of medication, or suffer from any illness or disease, before you begin an exercise routine.

Dehydration leads to increased HR. Long workouts, road races, and indoor workouts often lead to an increased HR at given workloads due to loss of total body water, primarily through sweating/evaporation.

Caffeine is found in many foodstuffs, and it is a stimulant to the central nervous system. The effect of any stimulant on the cardiovascular system is to increase both resting HR and average HR at any given workload. In excessive amounts, caffeine is considered a banned substance. Caffeine is also a diuretic, which means it increases urine output, and this can further encourage the onset of dehydration.

When an individual temporarily travels to altitude, atmospheric pressure decreases, and the cardiovascular system has to work harder to keep blood-oxygen levels within normal ranges. Ventilation increases, as do resting HR and exercise HR. These changes are most noticeable in the first week at altitude, and they are more pronounced with greater changes in elevation.

In hot environments, especially during sustained exercise, core temperature increases. The cardiovascular system has to work harder trying to keep the body cool. Because of this, exercise HR is significantly higher than in cooler environments. When exercise HR increases over time without a corresponding increase in effort, the physiological term is "cardiac drift." This occurs during long-duration exercise (longer than two hours) and high-humidity conditions (evaporative cooling through sweating is impaired), and dehydration is a contributing factor. Fluid loss decreases the plasma volume of your blood, which means that less blood is leaving your heart each time it beats. Since your body still needs the same amount of oxygenated blood, your heart must beat more frequently.

All of us deal with the stresses of life on a daily basis. In fact, exercise is one type of stress. So, just like during exercise, or any of the other variables already mentioned, our resting HR will increase during times of increased life stress. In fact, individuals with full and busy lives are at greater risk for overreaching or overtraining than those who have relatively simple lives, even though their total training time may be the same or less than that of others.

HOW TO TRAIN WITH POWER

Because of all the reasons just described, HR may not be the best method for prescribing intensity. Fortunately, other methods exist, and the method gaining in popularity most recently is the use of power. Power-measuring devices have become both commercially available and cost-effective for most cyclists in the last few years. Models from Powertap, SRM, and Polar can be mounted directly onto your bike and provide accurate real-time data. I predict that we'll see the day when powermeters are as widely used as, or even more widely used than, HR monitors.

Power is equal to work divided by a specific time period, and in cycling the unit of measurement for power is the watt. Power can also be defined as force times velocity. In the example of a cyclist, we are specifically referring to force at the pedal and the velocity of the legs or cadence. So, if your cadence remains constant, power increases if force at the pedal increases (or, if forces at the pedal decrease with a constant cadence, power decreases). To keep this simple, all you really need to know is that power is directly related to cycling performance. The more power you can generate for any given length of time, the better your ability.

Power can be utilized for prescribing exercise intensity in much the same way that we use HR monitors now. According to Dean Golich, one of our premier CTS coaches, "The use of power to prescribe training intensities works best for developing the specific energy systems, and I can do this in a much more logical and accurate way than by attempting to use a heart rate monitor alone." Ideally, with all athletes that CTS and I work with, intensity is prescribed using a combination of power as the primary indicator of intensity and HR as the secondary indicator. For longer, relatively low-intensity efforts, such as long (30 or more minutes) Tempos, I use both power and heart rate. However, for short-duration, high-intensity efforts, we will use power exclusively as the intensity measure, especially for anaerobic efforts, where the HR response isn't applicable.

Just like with average HR data from a CTS Field Test, we can also determine various power ranges from average power data:

Sample Field Test Results		
	EFFORT #1	EFFORT #2
Average Power	300 watts	290 watts

First, as opposed to taking the highest average HR from both efforts, we take the average power of both efforts together (assuming both efforts were of comparable quality). In this example, we get an initial average power output of 295 watts. However, if there is more than a 10 percent difference between Efforts #1 and #2, then we use the higher of the two.

Next, because we know that for a short-duration time trial, most cyclists can sustain a power output about 10 percent above LT, we decrease this number (295 watts) by 10 percent. Now our corrected value is approximately 265 watts, which should be within ±10 watts of LT power. By adding and subtracting 10 watts from the corrected power value, we calculate a wattage range of between 255 and 275 watts, which corresponds to this cyclist's SteadyState Interval.

Adjust the SS power range up by 10 percent to get your Climbing-Repeat (CR) range, and adjust the range down by 15 percent to get your Tempo (T) power range. Other specific workouts, such as RR, FM, and EM, use heart rate exclusively.

Describing the process for specific determination of critical powers for short, anaerobic efforts is beyond the scope of this book, but you can come reasonably close to estimating your own by simply performing two or three efforts of the specific duration you are looking for. Perform this test when you are well-rested, then average your power outputs to come up with a target power to achieve during future workouts. When you are no longer able to hit this target power during intervals, your workout is over. This is one of the big advantages of using a powermeter for anaerobic workouts. When your power output falls below 95 percent of your target, you are too fatigued to get any benefit from further intervals. You've done as much as you can do for that day, and anything more will just lead to increased fatigue.

Factors Affecting Power Output

Just like HR, many factors affect a cyclist's ability to produce power. Briefly, anything that compromises the body's ability to function efficiently usually also negatively impacts your ability to produce sustained power. Fortunately, power responds instantaneously to changes in workload. As the workload increases, power goes up; as the workload decreases, power goes down. Therefore, there is no lag time with respect to power. This makes power a highly sensitive indicator for determining training/recovery status, and you should continue with a prescribed session, or revise or postpone a session, based on your ability or inability to produce power.

CTS WORKOUTS

What follows are complete descriptions of all the workouts used in the training plans that appear elsewhere in this book. These are the same workouts I use with my athletes, and the same workouts all CTS coaches use with CTS members. Each workout is defined, and then further described in relation to the five training components introduced in Chapter Three. There are also instructions on how to properly perform each workout. The workouts are listed alphabetically, not necessarily in the order in which they should appear in a training plan.

ClimbingRepeats™ (CR)

These are similar to SS, except they are performed while climbing. CR improve your sustained climbing power. Your heart rate while climbing is slightly higher than what is seen on flat ground due to the increased muscle recruitment required for riding uphill. As a result, the CR heart rate range is closer to your time trial heart rate than your SS heart rate is. If you don't have access to a long steady climb, these efforts can be performed on an indoor trainer with the front wheel elevated 2 to 4 inches above the horizontal. Intervals can be 10 to 25 minutes long with 5 to 15 minutes recovery between efforts.

1. Intensity: 95 percent (under 35 years old) and 92 percent (Master) of average heart rate from CTS Field Test
2. Volume: 2 to 4, 8 to 20 minute efforts with 1:1 work recovery
3. Frequency: Allow at least 48 to 72 hours between sessions.
4. Terrain: Long steady climb
5. Pedal Cadence: 70 to 85 RPM

Goal: Increase your sustainable climbing power by training at the edge of your lactate threshold.

How to do it: This workout should be performed on the road with a long steady climb. The training intensity is based on your CTS Field Test, as calculated above. It is critical that you maintain this intensity for the length of the CR. Pedal cadence for CR intervals while climbing should be 70–85 RPM. Maintaining the training intensity is the most important factor, not pedal cadence. It is very important to avoid interruptions while doing these intervals. Focus on continuous riding for the length of the interval. Recovery time between the CR is equal to the length of the preceding interval.

DescendingIntervals™ (DI)

These are best performed indoors, even if the weather is good, primarily because of the complex nature of the workout. Only perform these maximal efforts after you are confident in the amount of time spent developing your aerobic energy systems. Pay attention to your perceived level of exertion, being sure you achieve a maximal effort each time. Adjust the number of sets and the length of the intervals according to your fitness and training needs. It is important to allow a minimum of two days of recovery between DI training days. These are short, maximal efforts, so heart-rate intensity is not prescribed.

1. Intensity: Maximal efforts
2. Volume: 2 to 3 sets with 5 to 7 efforts per set; 10 to 15 minutes recovery between sets.
3. Frequency: Allow at least 48 hours between sessions.
4. Terrain: Flat, or on an indoor trainer
5. Cadence: 110 or more rpm

Goal: To increase anaerobic power, lactate tolerance, and repeatability during short, intense efforts.

How to do it: This workout should be performed on an indoor trainer, because the controlled environment offers a better comparison from one session to another. It can also be performed on a relatively flat section of road. The gearing should be moderate and pedal cadence must be high (110 or higher) during each interval, and rpm takes precedence over gearing. Attack the start of each interval as explosively as possible. Jump out of the saddle as you begin the interval and attempt to build speed as the interval continues. If you have to, shift into a lighter gear to maintain the cadence, but don't let the intensity of the interval drop. With a high cadence, your heart rate will remain extremely high and you will train your muscles for high power and repeatability. Recovery between intervals is easy spinning. Recovery time between efforts is limited so that you will never fully recover between intervals. Heart rate intensity is not prescribed, because the interval is a maximal effort of relatively short duration. The recovery time between intervals is the same length as the maximal effort of the interval. Recovery time between DI sets is ten minutes, and you should eventually be able to do two to three sets total.

Here is an example of a DI workout:

One set consists of the following efforts and recovery intervals:

- 120 seconds at maximal effort followed by 120 seconds of recovery spinning
- 105 seconds at maximal effort followed by 105 seconds of recovery spinning
- 90 seconds at maximal effort followed by 90 seconds of recovery spinning
- 75 seconds at maximal effort followed by 75 seconds of recovery spinning
- 60 seconds at maximal effort followed by 60 seconds of recovery spinning
- 45 seconds at maximal effort followed by 45 seconds of recovery spinning
- 30 seconds at maximal effort followed by 30 seconds of recovery spinning

EnduranceMiles™ (EM)

An extension of the FM. The heart rate ceiling is slightly higher than during the FM. These workouts continue to develop the aerobic energy system, which, again, is the foundation of the CTS training philosophy. Just like the volume of the FM, adjust the volume of these workouts to meet the demands of your goals and your available training time. Using the slightly higher heart rate ceiling provides more flexibility, and EM are great for group rides. It is acceptable for the heart rate to increase a bit as long as 95 percent of the ride is spent below this prescribed ceiling.

1. Intensity: 91 percent (under 35 years old) and 88 percent (Master) of average heart rate from the CTS Field Test
2. Volume: appropriate for your goals and schedule; will increase as you progress through the Preparation Period
3. Frequency: Allow at least 18 hours between sessions.

4. Terrain: Flat to rolling
5. Pedal cadence: 85 to 95 rpm for experienced cyclists; if you are new to the sport, your range should be 95 or more rpm.

Goal: This is the next step after FoundationMiles. EM focus on building an aerobic energy system that will increase your endurance capabilities. Expected benefits include:

- Slow-twitch muscle fibers gain size and strength
- Increased capillary development
- Produces more mitochondria (muscle-cell structures that produce ATP)
- Increased stroke volume from your heart
- Improved temperature regulation
- Increased respiratory endurance

How to do it: This workout is used throughout the year. The pace during the EM workout is slightly quicker, and at a higher heart rate than the FM workout. Use your gearing as you hit the hills to remain in the saddle as you climb. Expect to keep your pedal speed up into the 85-to-95-rpm range.

FastPedal™ (FP)

FastPedal helps increase pedaling efficiency, allows you to widen your range of optimal cadences, and allows you to develop a smooth pedal stroke. Effective technique requires you to apply pressure through the entire pedal stroke, pulling through the bottom and over the top.

1. Intensity: not applicable; heart rate will climb during intervals, but it should not be used as indicator of intensity.
2. Volume: one to five efforts of 5 to 12 minutes each. Allow for equal durations of work and recovery.
3. Frequency: Allow at least 24 hours between sessions.
4. Terrain: Flat to slightly downhill; stationary trainers or rollers
5. Pedal cadence: 105 to 130+ rpm. Less-experienced cyclists may need to start at a slightly lower cadence range and then progress to higher cadences as technique improves.

Goal: Improves efficient pedaling mechanics through high-speed pedaling.

How to do it: This workout should be performed on a relatively flat section of road. The gearing should be light with low pedal resistance. Begin slowly increasing your pedal speed, starting out with about 15 or 16 pedal revolutions per ten-second count. This equates to a cadence of between 90 and 96 rpm. While staying in the saddle, further increase your pedal speed, keeping your hips steady with no rocking. Concentrate on pulling through the bottom of the pedal stroke and over the top. After two minutes of FastPedal, you should be maintaining between 18 and 22 pedal revolutions per ten-second count, or a cadence of between 108 and 130 rpm. Sustain your cadence for the rest of the interval. Your heart rate will climb while you do this workout, but don't use it to judge your training intensity. It is important that you try to ride the entire length of the FastPedal workout with as few interruptions as possible, since it should consist of continuous riding. If you find it difficult to perform this outdoors, try doing the first few sessions on a stationary trainer. If riding indoors, place some mirrors in strategic locations so you can obtain some immediate visual feedback. Do your best to avoid any bouncing and rocking of your hips.

FixedGear™ (FG)

This type of training helps to improve pedaling mechanics and efficiency, as well as to increase leg speed and strength. This is also an excellent way to maximize your training time, especially on cold days. The mechanics of a fixed-gear bike require you to pedal continuously. As long as the bike is moving forward, you have to pedal. FG training may be new to some of you, so I recommend that inexperienced riders use the fixed-gear bike on a stationary trainer for the first couple of rides.

1. Intensity: Dictated by terrain
2. Volume: 60 to 120 minutes
3. Frequency: Allow at least 18 hours between sessions. This will be dictated by time in the weight room.
4. Terrain: Flat to rolling
5. Pedal cadence: Dictated by terrain

Goal: Riding a fixed-gear bike has benefits that many elite cyclists enjoy.

- Smoother and better pedal mechanics
- Leg speed
- Leg strength

How to do it: Setting your bike up as a fixed-gear bike means you have no choice in gearing and pedaling (other than the initial setup). The fact that you have to pedal continuously develops a smooth pedal stroke as you spin down hills and increases leg strength as you grind up hills. Gearing is usually described by the ratio of chainring teeth to cog teeth. For instance, riding a 39×16 means your chain is sitting on a 39-tooth chainring in the front and a 16-tooth cog in the back. Generally, gearing for a fixed-gear bike will be light (42×19, 36×16), since this helps balance the gearing for various types of terrain. To make the gear bigger (more difficult to spin), move to a chainring with more teeth and/or a cog with fewer teeth. To make the gear smaller (easier to spin), move to a chainring with fewer teeth and/or a cog with more teeth. By no means do you have to go out and buy a bike specifically for this purpose. Use an old road bike, find a used fixed-gear rear wheel, and simply unthread your chain from the rear derailleur, shorten it, and place it around the small chain ring and the rear cog, and you're done. You can also use a track bike for this purpose; just be sure to install at least one brake before you go out on the road. Since this training is normally done during the Foundation Period, you are also possibly lifting weights. In order to train properly, you need to reduce one as you increase the other. A fixed-gear bike allows greater aerobic benefits with less time on the bike, so you can spend more time in the weight room.

FoundationMiles™ (FM)

As the name implies, this is the groundwork for all future training. FM builds the aerobic engine and prepares the body for future high-intensity training. Lighter (lower) gears and slightly higher cadences (85 to 95 rpm) lead to size and strength gains in slow-twitch muscle fibers, development of capillary and mitochondrial structures, and a decrease in resting heart rate. Your goals for total ride time are based on your training goals and current fitness level. There should be a progressive increase in volume as training progresses from one week to the next and from one month to the next. Focus on developing the aerobic system and proper pedaling mechanics. I like to prescribe FastPedal as part of FM workouts. The lower heart rate ceiling also keeps you from working too hard on the bike, if you are incorporating resistance training into your training program.

1. Intensity: 89 percent (under 35 years old) and 86 percent (Master) of average heart rate from a CTS Field Test
2. Volume: Appropriate for your goals and available time for training; increase gradually as you progress through the Foundation Period.
3. Frequency: Allow at least 18 hours between sessions.
4. Terrain: Flat to rolling
5. Pedal cadence: 85 to 95 rpm for experienced cyclists; if you are new to the sport, your range should be 95+ rpm

Goal: This is the cornerstone workout for your endurance training. FM prepares your aerobic system for the physical adaptations that will be developed later through other forms of more intense training. Expected benefits include:

- Slow-twitch muscle fibers gain size and strength.
- Increases capillary development
- Increases the number of mitochondria
- Decreases resting heart rate

How to do it: This workout is not necessarily limited to the Foundation Period. I recommend that you incorporate FM workouts into your training year-round. As mentioned previously, all riding below the prescribed heart rate ceiling involves your aerobic energy system, and the goal is not to exceed this ceiling. Again, if you find the relative lack of structure for FM boring, then add some FP within the prescribed FM time.

HighSpeedSprints™ (HSS)

These are great workouts to help develop the ability to be there for the "endgame" of field sprinting. HSS can be done with a partner, perhaps with you and your partner alternating at the leadout position. It is also important to allow for full recovery after each HSS effort; otherwise you won't be able to put forth a maximal effort for subsequent efforts. Heart rate response will lag behind the effort, so it isn't necessary to adhere to any heart rate range for these efforts.

1. Intensity: Maximal efforts with start speed of 30 to 35 MPH
2. Volume: between four and eight efforts of 8 to 12 seconds each, with 10 to 20 minutes recovery between efforts
3. Frequency: Allow at least 48 hours between sessions.
4. Terrain: Slight downhill
5. Cadence: 110+ rpm

Goal: HSS develops your top-end power and speed. This type of sprinting improves your peak power. Since it is performed slightly downhill at high speed and high pedal cadence, the power demands will be huge due to the aerodynamic drag associated with beginning sprints at high speed.

How to do it: Sprints are always performed at maximum output. On a slight downhill, you should be rolling along at a high speed (30 to 35 mph, depending on your level of development) in a large gear. Jump out of the saddle, and accelerate. Upon reaching top speed, return to the saddle and focus on holding your top speed for the length of the sprint interval. Maintain good form and focus on maintaining high pedal speed with smooth and efficient form for the entire sprint. These sprints should be 8 to 12 seconds in length. Full recovery between sprints allows muscles to rebuild ATP and ensures a quality sprint workout. Normally, 10 to 20 minutes allows for enough recovery between HSS efforts. Pedal speed is high for these sprints: 110+ rpm.

MuscleTension Intervals™ (MT)

This is another excellent way to convert strength gains from the weight room into power on the bicycle. MT assists with the recruitment of fast-twitch muscle fibers. Avoid including this exercise in your training regime if you have chronic knee problems, or at the very least, use lighter gears and a slightly higher cadence. Intervals can range in duration from 5 to 15 minutes, with 5 to 10 minutes of rest between efforts. The MT efforts do not induce a high heart-rate response, so there is no need for a HR target range and recovery does not need to be long.

1. Intensity: This is a muscular workout, so heart rate is not a good indicator of intensity and should remain low. Gearing will dictate intensity: 53×12–15
2. Volume: Two to four efforts of 5 to 12 minutes each, with recoveries of half the duration of the efforts.
3. Frequency: Allow at least 48 hours between sessions.
4. Terrain: Uphill (5 to 8% grade)
5. Pedal cadence: 50 to 55 rpm

Goal: To develop cycling-specific strength. High muscle tension during the intervals assists in the recruitment of fast-twitch muscle fibers, which are important during intense efforts.

How to do it: This workout should be performed on a long, moderate climb or on a trainer with your front wheel raised 2 to 4 inches above the normal horizontal plane to let you simulate your climbing position. Pedal cadence must be low (50 to 55 rpm) and heart rate intensity is not important, because this is primarily a muscular exercise when performed correctly. Large gears (such as 53×12–15 uphill) are required to produce the low cadence and high muscle tension. Correct form must be strictly maintained during these intervals. Strong concentration is needed to keep your upper body absolutely steady and relaxed while concentrating on correct pedaling form (exerting force over the top and through the bottom of the pedal stroke). If you are monitoring your HR during these efforts, and it begins to enter your Tempo range, you are most likely riding at too high an intensity level. Additionally, if you find that your legs start to feel like they are burning or loading up, especially within the first few minutes, then again, you are performing the efforts at too high an intensity level.

OverUnder Intervals™ (OU)

This workout requires 24 to 48 hours of recovery, depending on the length of the intervals. Adjust the length of time at and above lactate threshold based on your level of fitness and physical development. Recovery will also be based on your level of fitness.

1. Intensity: There are two—SS heart rate range and CR heart rate range.
2. Volume: Two to six total efforts per set, with efforts consisting of 5 to 10 minutes at SS and then two to three minutes above SS. 5 to 10 minutes of recovery between efforts.
3. Frequency: One day per week
4. Terrain: Flat, or on an indoor trainer
5. Cadence: 100 to 115 rpm

Goal: To develop lactate tolerance and buffering capability in order to build power at intensities just above lactate threshold.

How to do it: This workout should be performed on a relatively flat section of road or on an indoor trainer. The gearing should be moderate, and pedal cadence should be high (100 rpm or higher). Slowly bring your intensity up to your SS HR range. Maintain this heart rate intensity for five minutes, then increase your heart rate intensity to CR HR range. Hold this intensity for approximately half the time you spent at SS intensity, then drop your intensity back to your SS HR range. You will continue this pattern of riding in your SteadyState range, increasing your intensity, and then returning to your SteadyState range, as your ability allows. A typical set equals: SS/CR/SS/CR/SS/CR, then recovery.

This workout builds up high levels of lactic acid. Working in this way trains your body to dissipate and buffer lactate, also known as increasing your lactate tolerance. Normally you should limit the length of the interval above lactate threshold to two to three minutes, while the intervals at lactate threshold are normally five to ten minutes long. Lactate threshold training is very stressful on the body and needs to be performed with great care. When in doubt, perform fewer efforts, and limit yourself to 2 sets.

PowerIntervals™ (PI)

These are particularly good when you aren't racing or competing much. These are maximal efforts, so the heart rate should be above your CR heart rate range. PI efforts develop maximal aerobic capacity, and this will be reflected by an increase in your VO_2max.

1. Intensity: Maximal
2. Volume: Three to eight efforts of 3 to 5 minutes each, with the ratio of work to recovery at between 1:1 and 1:1.5. The efforts can be divided into sets.
3. Frequency: Allow at least 36 hours between sessions, depending on your level of development and whether or not you are racing.
4. Terrain: Flat, or on an indoor trainer
5. Pedal cadence: 110 to 120+ rpm; maintain the cadence throughout the effort.

Goal: To increase power output during short, intense efforts.

How to do it: This workout is best performed on an indoor trainer, because the controlled environment allows for better comparison from one session to another. It can also be performed on a relatively flat section of road. The gearing should be moderate, but pedal cadence must be high (110 rpm or higher), and cadence takes precedence over gear selection. Take one minute to build up to a maximum effort, and then maintain this intensity for the remaining interval. The last two minutes of each interval is what develops your maximum aerobic capacity. If you have to, shift into a lighter gear to maintain the cadence, but don't let the intensity of the interval drop. With a high cadence, your heart rate will remain extremely high and you will train your body's ability to deliver oxygen to the muscles. Recovery between intervals is easy spinning.

Lance Armstrong and George Hincapie are among the athletes who use this interval session. Since the addition of this workout to Lance and George's training programs, I have seen them further develop their extraordinary ability to attack on steep hills late in races when everyone else is gasping for air.

PowerStart™ (PS)

These are designed to develop and train the ATP/PC energy system. PS efforts are short, maximal bursts of 8 to 12 seconds with complete recovery (five to ten minutes), so the ATP levels can be restored. The gear needs to be relatively large (52–53×12–16), depending on your level of development, but if it is too big, you won't be able to generate enough power to properly execute the workout. Because the efforts are so short, there isn't a target HR range to consider.

1. Intensity: Maximal
2. Volume: 4 to 12 efforts of 8 to 12 seconds each. These can be divided into sets of two to four efforts per set. Since these are maximal efforts, you need to allow for full recovery between them.
3. Frequency: Allow at least 36 hours between sessions.
4. Terrain: Flat, but the workout could be performed on a gradual slope to develop additional pedal force.
5. Pedal cadence: Not applicable (see below)

Goal: To increase your power delivery to the pedals; these workouts help convert gains made through resistance training in the gym to the bike.

How to do it: This workout should be performed on a relatively flat section of road. The gearing should be very large, depending on your level of physical development. The PowerStart should begin at a very low speed—a near-standstill. Jump up out of the saddle, driving the pedals down as hard as possible. Perform the entire exercise out of the saddle, and make every attempt to keep your upper body stationary as you progress through the effort. The PowerStart should not last longer than ten pedal strokes or 12 seconds. This is a muscular workout, and heart rate will not have time to respond. Also, since you are starting from a

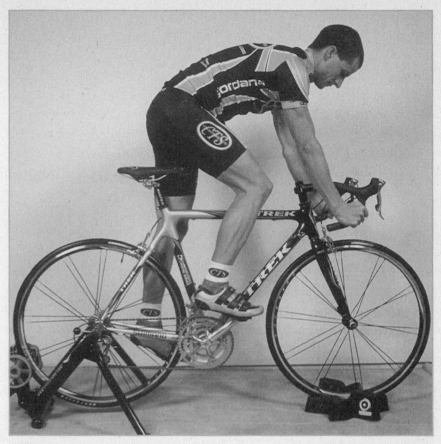

CTS Coach Jim Lehman demonstrating proper starting position for PowerStart. *Photo © by Charlie Lengal III*

standing start, there is no cadence range. By the time the effort is over, you should feel as if you are just getting on top of the gear.

RaceSimulation™ (RS)

This is an effective way to make use of all the hard group rides. It prepares you physically and mentally for the demands of racing, and it reinforces the need to be alert while riding in the bunch. RaceSimulation helps new and experienced cyclists to develop tactical awareness. It is important to limit the amount of RS you participate in because of the elevated intensity and stress. Allow for adequate recovery following these workouts. If the RS was less than two hours, you can train on the day following an RS workout, but I generally limit workouts to aerobic intensities. If the RS was more than two hours, I usually recommend that the following day be a rest day.

1. Intensity: As dictated by ride
2. Volume: 15 to 120 minutes. Increase the volume as you progress through periodization.
3. Frequency: One day per week if you are racing, two days per week if not
4. Terrain: As dictated by ride; look for a group ride that mimics the terrain of your upcoming events.
5. Cadence: 80 to 110 rpm

Goal: This workout simulates the demands that occur in races. You will be using all your energy systems to maintain the intensity of the workout.

How to do it: This workout is best performed during a club or group ride. Riding with a group tends to push you to new heights of intensity and simulates the demands of racing. During the ride, there should be a series of accelerations followed by slower riding; sudden attacks; increasing tempo on climbs; and random attacks and counterattacks. Generally, you should not participate in a large volume of RS training. Since this simulates a race situation, you will need plenty of recovery time following one of these workouts. I usually prescribe this type of training year-round, not just during the Specialization Period. During the Preparation Period, keep the length of the RS training short—between 15 and 60 minutes. Pedal cadence should match that of a race: 80 to 110 rpm, depending on the terrain and intensity.

RecoveryRide™ (RR)

A vital part of every training program, RR should be used throughout the training year. Without rides such as these, coupled with rest days, the body cannot adapt to the demands of training. Adaptation to training occurs during rest and recovery, NOT when you are actually training.

This is an excellent opportunity for you to ride with your spouse, significant other, and/or child. Make it a relaxing ride, both mentally and physically. Often, unwise cyclists believe that these rides are too easy and end up going harder than they should, particularly as fitness level increases. Don't make the same mistake that they do.

1. Intensity: 65 to 70 percent of average heart rate from a CTS Field Test
2. Volume: 30 to 120 minutes, depending on your level of development. The more volume and/or intensity, the longer the RR should be.
3. Frequency: At least once a week, more often during regeneration weeks
4. Terrain: Flat
5. Pedal cadence: 75 to 85 rpm

Goal: To speed the recovery process by riding at an easy pace at low resistance on flat terrain. Benefits include: increasing blood flow to the muscles to help relieve muscle soreness and reduce free-radical buildup that causes muscle stress and damage. Studies have shown that active recovery leads to faster recovery than complete rest.

How to do it: Recovery rides should be between 30 and 120 minutes in duration on flat terrain. Keep your cadence lower than normal, staying in a light gear to keep resistance low. Heart rate must also remain low, even if you hit any hills; just slow down and use your gears to keep the resistance low. The key to recovery rides is to ride just enough to engage the active recovery process, but not long or intensely enough to induce a training stress.

SpeedIntervals™ (SI)

These are excellent for preparing you for the demands of criterium racing and are utilized exclusively during the Specialization Period. SI can be 30 to 50 seconds long with equal recovery periods. You should focus on maintaining a high cadence, so it is not necessary to prescribe a heart-rate range for these workouts. It is important to maintain proper form during these efforts. If your pedal stroke becomes sloppy or your form begins to deteriorate, it is time to stop the workout. These are very demanding workouts, so it is important to pay close attention to the signs of overtraining when you are doing a block of SI.

1. Intensity: Maximal efforts; the intensity is dictated by the cadence.
2. Volume: 6 to 24, efforts of 30 to 50 seconds each with a 1:1 work-to-recovery ratio; the efforts can be divided into sets.
3. Frequency: Allow at least 48 hours between sessions.
4. Terrain: Flat to slightly downhill
5. Pedal cadence: 110 to 130 rpm, specific to a goal event, so you may need to increase your pedal cadence as your goal approaches.

Goal: To develop repeatable speed and power.

How to do it: This workout should be performed on a relatively flat section of road with a slight tailwind to enhance your top speed during the efforts. The gearing should be moderate, but pedal cadence must be high (110 or higher), and again, like PI efforts, cadence takes precedence over gearing. Speed, power, and accelerations, not heart rate, are the key elements. This workout builds up high levels of lactic acid and trains your body to dissipate and buffer lactate. You should limit the length of each interval to one minute or less. If you have to, shift into a lighter gear to maintain the cadence, but don't let the intensity of the interval drop. With a high cadence, you will train your body's ability to perform repeated high-speed efforts. Recovery between intervals is easy spinning. Recovery time between SI efforts is limited in order to build repeatability. Speed training is very stressful to the body and needs to be performed with great care. During the weeks when you perform SI efforts, you need to reduce your overall training hours to encourage recovery.

SteadyState Intervals™ (SS)

These are designed to improve your ability to produce power at lactate threshold. By training slightly below lactate threshold, you develop the capacity to work harder without increasing blood-lactate levels above resting levels. This capacity develops as the body becomes more efficient at clearing lactate as the muscles produce it. As a result of this training adaptation, you can produce more power at a given heart rate, which is essential for cycling success. It is better to err on the conservative side when establishing a heart-rate range for these workouts. Spending too much time at or above lactate threshold can be very taxing and will ultimately diminish any gains you are attempting to achieve.

1. Intensity: 92 percent (under 35 years old) and 90 percent (Master) of the average heart rate from a CTS Field Test, plus two to four beats per minute.
2. Volume: Two to four efforts of 8 to 20 minutes each, with a 1:1 work-to-recovery ratio
3. Frequency: Allow at least 48 hours between sessions.
4. Terrain: Flat to rolling
5. Pedal cadence: 85 to 95 rpm; specific to a goal event, so you may need to increase your pedal cadence as your goals approach.

Goal: To increase your lactate threshold by training at the edge of your lactate threshold.

How to do it: This workout can either be performed on the road with a long steady climb, on hills, or on flat terrain. The training intensity is based on your CTS Field Test, as calculated above. It is critical that you maintain this intensity for the length of the interval. Interruptions during the interval limit the adaptations from this workout. Pedal cadence for SS Intervals on short hills should be 70 to 80 rpm, and flat-terrain cadence should be 85 to 95 rpm. Maintaining the appropriate intensity, NOT the pedal cadence, is the most important factor. Focus on continuous riding for the length of the prescribed interval. SteadyState Intervals are meant to be done at slightly below your individual time trial pace, so don't make the mistake of riding at your time trial pace during them.

Stomps™ (S)

These are designed to improve muscular strength and power while in the saddle. Stomps should be 15 to 20 seconds in length, with at least five minutes of rest between efforts. This workout is another excellent way to convert strength gains made in the weight room to strength and power on the bike. As you gain strength, you can increase the resistance by decreasing the starting speed.

1. Intensity: Maximal
2. Volume: 4 to 12, efforts of 15 to 20 seconds each. They can be divided into sets. Since these are maximal efforts, you need to allow for full recovery between them.
3. Frequency: Allow at least 36 hours between sessions.
4. Terrain: Flat to slightly downhill
5. Pedal cadence: Not applicable (see below)

Goal: To increase muscular power at the pedal while remaining seated.

How to do it: This workout should be performed on a relatively flat section of road with a slight tailwind. The gearing should be large, 53×12 (depending on your level of physical development, much like PS). The effort should begin at a moderate speed (typically 15 to 20 mph); then, while seated in the saddle, begin to STOMP the pedals as hard as possible! Concentrate on pulling through the bottom of the pedal stroke and smoothly stomping down during the downstroke. Keep your upper body as still as possible and let your legs drive the pedals. The Stomps should last 15 to 20 seconds each, with at least five minutes of recovery between efforts. This is a muscular workout, and heart rate may not have time to respond.

Tempo™ (T)

This enhances and develops the upper-end aerobic system, thus allowing you to produce the majority of your power aerobically. This workout lays the groundwork for future high-intensity workouts. Make sure that your Tempo workouts are performed without disruption—i.e., traffic signals, dangerous intersections, stop signs, etc. If uninterrupted Tempo workouts are not possible, then perform them indoors. Typically, I expect my elite-level riders to be able to perform a 120-minute Tempo effort without much difficulty, and my recreational riders should be able to complete a 45-minute Tempo.

1. Intensity: 88 percent (under 35 years old) and 87 percent (Master) of the average heart rate from a CTS Field Test, plus two to four beats per minute
2. Volume: 20 to 120 minutes of continuous riding
3. Frequency: Allow at least 36 hours between sessions, depending on your level of development.
4. Terrain: Flat to rolling
5. Pedal cadence: 70 to 75 rpm

Goal: Strategically placing Tempo workouts into your training program has many advantages:

- Greater comfort while cruising on rolling terrain
- Better fuel utilization during long races or rides
- Increased capacity for more intense workouts
- Better power at moderate intensities
- Increased muscle glycogen storage capacity
- Improved free fatty acid oxidation, which spares muscle glycogen
- Increased development of mitochondria
- Improved aerobic efficiency

How to do it: Pedal cadence should be low. Try a 70- to 75-rpm range while staying at the prescribed heart rate intensity. This helps to increase pedal resistance and strengthens leg muscles. Also, try to stay in the saddle when you hit hills during your Tempo workouts. This adds more pedal resistance and readies the connective tissues and supporting muscle groups before your training heads into more explosive workouts. It is important that you try to ride the entire length of the Tempo workout with as few interruptions as possible; to achieve maximum benefit, Tempo workouts should consist of continuous riding.

FLEXIBILITY

Your range of motion, or ability to move a joint or group of joints comfortably from one endpoint to another, can be defined as flexibility. Your ability to produce power, comfortably maintain your cycling position, and optimally control your bicycle can be affected by your flexibility. Many overuse injuries develop originally because of general inflexibility and/or flexibility imbalances between opposing muscle groups. Lack of flexibility can ultimately lead to many problems, particularly with the knees, hamstrings, and lower back. Stretching preserves and enhances your flexibility and is a vital part of training for all cyclists.

There are three types of stretching: ballistic, static, and proprioceptive neuromuscular facilitation (PNF). Ballistic stretching requires a bouncing motion on the part of the athlete. I don't recommend this type of stretching for any reason, because the risk of injury is high. PNF stretching requires the assistance of a partner, and because of the increased complexity, it is usually not appropriate for the individual athlete. Static stretching is my method of choice. Static stretching simply requires you to slowly stretch a muscle group or joint to its farthest point (defined by the point of increased resistance to further stretch and the onset of slight discomfort) and then to maintain this stretch for as little as 10 seconds or as long as 30 seconds or more.

Stretching is most effective when muscles are warm. Thus, post-exercise stretching is the best way to improve flexibility. Alternatively, if you know you are generally inflexible or have experienced overuse injuries in the past, you may also want to stretch before the primary workout begins, but also after you have warmed up at a relatively low intensity (RR) for 10 to 20 minutes. However, most of us have limited time available for training, and, at the end of a workout, time is often not available for stretching. Another suggestion is to stretch in the evening while watching TV. I suggest that you take a long, hot shower or bath to help warm the muscles before you begin.

Specific recommendations for your stretching routine appear on page 115]. Due to the infinite number of stretches and variations available, I suggest that you determine your own stretches, based on the muscle groups and joints that you perceive to be the most inflexible. At a minimum, be sure to address the major muscle groups (quadriceps, hamstrings, abdomen, low back, chest, neck, upper back). Add or remove stretches as your training dictates. If in doubt, you may want to pursue the suggestions of a fitness professional.

Stretching Routine Recommendations

TYPE	STATIC
Stretches	All major muscle groups at a minimum, 4–6 total
Intensity	Low
Degree of Stretch	To endpoint of range of motion
Frequency	Three times per week at a minimum
Repetitions	One or two per stretch, depending on time available
Duration	Hold each stretch for 10–30 seconds.
Movement Speed	Slow
Time	Ideally, immediately after a workout; alternatively, after initial warmup, before primary workout

RECOVERY

The longer I am involved in coaching, the more evident it becomes that most cyclists underutilize or, even worse, totally ignore recovery as a tool that facilitates effective training. It is best to think of recovery as part of your training and to give it as high a priority as workouts and nutrition. I define recovery as anything and everything that assists an athlete's adaptation to training, with the exception of actual participation in the exercise session. RecoveryRides (RR); massage; nutrition before, during, and after a workout; and stretching are all examples of recovery techniques. The more recovery techniques you can consistently integrate into your training, the better.

As I have mentioned previously, it is in the time between races, and between workout sessions, that your adaptations to training occur. Your ability to "bridge the gap" between potentially excessive training and exceptional performance is determined by how well you implement and integrate any or all of the following recovery techniques. Ultimately, your ability to repeatedly perform at peak levels throughout the racing season is limited by how well your muscles recover and repair themselves after each race. Without adequate time for recovery, adaptation won't occur, and your development as a cyclist will be compromised.

I discussed the importance of active recovery when I described the RR workout. However, the more frequently you can incorporate some active recovery into your daily activities, the better. You don't need to wait until a scheduled RR to exploit the benefits of active recovery:

- Perform 20 to 30 minutes of RR after a hard group ride instead of getting into the car immediately afterward.
- Perform 30 to 45 minutes of RR after a race, and especially before an extended car trip to return home.
- If you are a competitive cyclist and you race in two separate categories, be sure to perform 30 to 45 minutes of RR immediately after your first race.
- If you have two high-intensity days scheduled back-to-back, perform 20 to 30 minutes of RR on your stationary trainer in the evening between the two days.
- If you work full-time and do most of your training in the evenings, try performing 20 to 30 minutes of RR each morning. If you train in the mornings, then allow 20 to 30 minutes of RR each evening.
- If you are incorporating resistance training into your plan, include 20 to 30 minutes of RR immediately after your resistance-training workout.

What Should You Do on the Days Between Races?

Full recovery between races may consist of a different protocol for each athlete, but the concept remains the same. You need to ride enough to stimulate active recovery but not enough to introduce a training load. The few days between races are not the time to pursue fitness goals. Simple rides of 30 to 120 minutes at a low heart rate and a comfortable pedal speed will aid recovery. For example, George Hincapie completed the following recovery riding after winning the 2001 Ghent-Wevelgem race, three days before the Paris-Roubaix World Cup race:

Thursday 18	75 minutes of easy spinning at 75–80 rpm, RecoveryMiles heart rate ceiling
Friday 19	60 minutes of easy spinning at 75–80 rpm, RecoveryMiles average heart rate ceiling
Saturday 20	Two hours at RecoveryMiles heart rate with two short high-power efforts of five minutes and two minutes of recovery between efforts

The riding he did was at low heart rates and low power outputs. This helped him to avoid inducing training stress, but it also helped speed the recovery process by increasing blood flow, accelerating the inflow of nutrients, and reducing muscle soreness. Additionally, the recovery riding helped him relax mentally by spending quiet time on the bike.

The day before Paris-Roubaix, George did two short efforts above lactate threshold (LT). This helped "open him up" and activated the clearance process of removing lactate. The inclusion of a few short, intense efforts the day before a race is useful in eliminating race-day sluggishness. Keep the efforts short (three to five minutes) and intense, and under no circumstances fatigue yourself.

Morning Heart Rate: Your Wake-Up Call

Monitoring resting heart rate is a valuable tool in gauging the recovery process and establishing individual recovery patterns. Monitoring resting (sleeping and morning) heart rate is so crucial that I occasionally have my athletes strap on a heart rate monitor as they sleep. Downloaded heart rate data from stage races or tough one-day races can then be used to assist in gauging recovery patterns. Generally, in a stage race an athlete's average sleeping heart rate will drop off by one to two beats per minute (bpm) each night. This pattern will continue for three to seven days, and normally after seven days his or her average sleeping heart rate will begin to rise by one to two bpm per night. While the average sleeping heart rate is dropping, the perceived effort during the race is rising. This is normally a tough time for the athlete, and his or her results may also drop off. Once the athlete's average sleeping heart rate begins to climb again, the perceived effort during the race generally becomes easier. This indicates that the athlete is beginning to adapt to the stress of stage racing and is getting stronger.

Keep your heart rate monitor next to the bed so you can quickly strap it on in the morning to check your morning heart rate. Take your morning heart rate before getting out of bed. Recording this heart rate data over a long period of time can help indicate heart rate trends that can be matched to a pattern of individual recovery. Look for lower and/ or higher morning heart rates that correspond to a greater perceived effort in your races or workouts. After a few months of recording this data, you should soon see trends in morning heart rate that can help you establish your individual recovery pattern.

10 Steps for Quicker Recovery

1. Make sure you begin to replenish depleted muscle-glycogen stores with high-glycemic-index carbohydrates within 30 minutes after completing a workout.
2. Make sure recovery rides between races and high-intensity workouts are only long enough to stimulate the active recovery process.
3. Select a sport drink with a carbohydrate-to-protein ratio of four grams of carbohydrate per gram of protein. This type of drink will maximally stimulate the insulin response in order to speed glycogen replenishment and the rebuilding of protein.
4. Power naps—take them as often as you can.
5. Limit the amount of protein and fat consumed in the immediate post-exercise period. Too much protein post-exercise hinders recovery by slowing hydration and carbohydrate replenishment. Again, the optimum ratio is four grams of carbohydrate per gram of protein.

6. Keep your riding intensity below 70 percent of your average HR from your Field Test results during RecoveryRides. This helps promote the recovery process by increasing blood flow and reducing muscle soreness without inducing fatigue.

7. Incorporate antioxidants into your nutrition program. Antioxidants can help protect against post-exercise muscle damage, thereby reducing the potential for soreness.

8. Drink fluids containing sodium, potassium, and magnesium during and following your races.

9. Massage. An extensive massage from a qualified massage therapist just once a month can make a noticeable difference. Self-massage is beneficial, too. Focusing on the legs, after a hot bath or shower, elevate one leg at a time against a wall or a piece of furniture, and begin at the ankles and gradually work your massage up the calf and then to the thigh. Spend about five minutes on each part, 20 minutes total. This can be performed daily.

10. Record your morning heart rate with a heart-rate monitor to begin establishing trends in your sleeping and morning heart rates. Use the changes in your morning HR to modify training as needed.

5

Going the Extra Mile

RESISTANCE TRAINING

Over the years, I have developed a very defined view of weight training. Cyclists benefit from resistance training, but weights and cycling don't mix well. Too often, I see amateur cyclists add resistance training to their programs without regard for the impact it will have on their training on the bike. Resistance training creates a substantial training load, and cyclists must compensate for that load by reducing the volume or intensity of their cycling training. The intensity and volume of your resistance training and aerobic training are inversely related: increased time in the gym means less time on the bike, and vice versa. With this in mind, by adhering to the following points, you can design a comprehensive training program that incorporates resistance training into your cycling program.

Understanding the Basics of Resistance Training for Cycling

Your resistance training program needs to address cycling-specific goals, especially if you want to see improvements in cycling strength, power, and endurance. I view resistance training as weight training coupled with on-the-bike resistance workouts. These on-bike workouts are essential for transforming strength gained in the gym into power delivered on the road.

I believe that the majority of resistance training should be done during the Foundation Period. The intensity of this period is generally low, making this the best time of year to balance the training loads from resistance and cycling training. Your resistance-training program needs to follow a periodization plan similar to the overall plan you have designed for the training year. In this case, you start with the Transition Phase before moving on to the Hypertrophy Phase, High-Volume Phase, Strength Phase, and Power Phase. Generally I try to confine the weight-training portion of an amateur cyclist's resistance-training program to 8 to 12 weeks, depending on the athlete's goals and experience level. During this period of time, weight training is the primary source of intensity in the athlete's program. Aerobic conditioning can still continue, but the intensity must be decreased to accommodate for the training load from the weight training. As the weight-training portion of the program tapers off, the frequency and volume of on-the-bike resistance-training workouts increases. These workouts include PowerStarts, Stomps, and MuscleTension.

NOTE: If this is your first year of resistance training, please concentrate on learning the proper technique of the exercises, and work in the range of 8 to 12 repetitions.

Transition Phase

The season is over and you've taken a few weeks of active rest, which means less time on the bike and the inclusion of other forms of aerobic training in order to maintain your fitness. This period is essential, since it helps prevent both physical and mental burnout. In most parts of the country, the days are also shorter and colder, and you're getting adjusted to regular indoor training.

Resistance training begins with a Transition Phase, not to be confused with the Transition Period of the annual periodization plan. The Transition Phase is a shift from a focus on cycling to an emphasis on strength training. The purpose is to prepare you for the higher-intensity resistance training that comes later. Just as you ease back into training on the bike or any type of aerobic exercise, you need to ease into strength training. The emphasis is on getting started correctly, without experiencing unnecessary muscle soreness.

A good way to ease yourself into resistance training is to perform exercises that utilize your body weight, including push-ups, pull-ups, abdominal crunches, floor back extensions, and lunges. You can also use light dumbbells to work the muscles in a similar fashion, especially if joint problems make push-ups or pull-ups uncomfortable.

There are two established training modes for weight training: circuit training and priority training. In circuit training, you perform a set of Exercise A, then go immediately to a set of Exercise B, then to a set of Exercise C, etc. until you have performed each movement. Circuit training is acceptable for the Transition Phase because it incorporates many exercises and allows you to get accustomed to the ranges of motion used in weightlifting. However, rest is minimal between exercises and exercises vary greatly, so the standard benefits of resistance training (strength, power, and muscular growth) are minimized. This is why you should use the priority-training mode of weight training for the majority of your resistance-training program.

In a priority-training workout, you perform a set of Exercise A, rest one to two minutes, perform another set of Exercise A, rest one to two minutes, and perform a third set of Exercise A. After this you will rest again, and prepare for the first set of Exercise B. Remember to actually step away from the exercise apparatus and move around between sets. Get a drink of water, record your workout in a training log, or cheer on your training partner during this break. You need to recover and come back ready for another hard effort on your next set.

During the Transition Phase of resistance training, and regardless of whether you are using circuit training or priority training, you should complete 12 to 15 repetitions (reps) for each of one to three sets of each exercise (i.e., each set contains 12 to 15 reps). Resistance is light-to-moderate. This phase is similar to your easy spinning, low-geared first attempt at winter riding outdoors. This phase usually lasts two to four weeks.

High-Volume Phase

Once you complete the two to four weeks of Transition Phase lifting, your training switches to increased resistance and fewer reps, and to a greater number of sets. In the High-Volume Phase, the weights are moderate, reps are 8 to 12 per set, and the number of sets is four to six. This phase is important, because you are preparing the muscles for the high-intensity resistance training to follow in the Strength Phase. This phase should coincide with your longer FM and EM rides, and may last between two and four weeks.

Strength Phase

Next, you will switch to a Strength Phase, where the object is to gain maximum strength. Heavier weights are used, 6 to 8 reps are performed per set, and the number of sets drops to three to five. Before lifting heavy weights it is essential to have a proper warmup, performing the same movement with lighter weights than you will be using during the actual strength workout.

This phase is similar to adding hard work to your riding. You need to complete Foundation Period training before you are ready for harder cycling workouts, and the same is true of weight training. The previous phases prepared your muscles and connective tissues for the stress of the Strength Phase. If you start the Strength Phase without properly training through the Transition and High-Volume Phases, you are likely to injure yourself. This phase also lasts between two and four weeks.

Power Development—"On-Bike Resistance Workouts"

At this point, you have arrived at the time of the season when you must begin putting more time in the saddle in order to maximize your aerobic engine. Resistance training is beneficial to a cyclist, but aerobic development is the cornerstone of your performance as an endurance athlete. You will continue to include resistance training as part of your workouts, but now it begins to take the form of on-the-bike resistance training. Strength gained in the gym is useless to you unless you can apply it to a cycling motion, and that's what PowerStarts, Stomps, and MuscleTension workouts can do. Using powermeters, I have found even more benefit from performing on-the-bike resistance-training workouts after weight training earlier in the same day. George Hincapie's peak power outputs for PowerStarts and Stomps are higher when he performs them in the afternoon after lifting weights in the morning.

Normally, I prescribe on-the-bike resistance training two to three times per week. It is important not to simply stop all resistance training so early that the benefits disappear by the time the big races or events arrive. A great deal of strength can be maintained with a minimal investment in training by including on-the-bike resistance training at least once a week. I also believe it is wise to maintain some maintenance strength work, especially in body parts like the abdominal muscles, the arms, and the back that do not receive as much stress as your legs through cycling.

Power workouts: On-the-bike workouts like PowerStarts, Stomps, and MuscleTension Intervals.

Periodized Weight Training

PHASE	DAYS/WEEK	SETS	REPETITIONS	WEIGHT	LENGTH
Transition	3	1–3	12–15	Light	2–4 weeks
Volume	3	4–6	8–12	Moderate	2–4 weeks
Strength	3	3–5	6–8	Heavy	2–4 weeks

Components of Effective Resistance Training

Frequency

Ideally, you should shoot for three resistance-training workouts per week, with at least one rest day between workouts. If you have less time available for training, you can also try two times per week, with at least two rest (i.e., no lifting) days after each resistance session.

Equipment Selection

Free weights are the best option available for resistance training. You have to use many muscles to balance and control free weights, in addition to the muscles you are primarily trying to develop. Developing those accessory muscles increases the integrity of your joints and helps prevent injury. The one disadvantage is that free weights may be less safe than machines and therefore require spotters for safety. Have a qualified training professional check that you have proper weightlifting technique before you progress beyond the Transition Phase of resistance training.

Exercise Selection

One of the simplest ways to ensure that you will develop a comprehensive resistance program is to divide your workout into the following five categories:

- Upper-body pushing
- Upper-body pulling
- Lower back
- Abdominals
- Lower body

You can perform one to two exercises from each of these categories with free weight or on machines.

UPPER-BODY PUSHING EXERCISES Upper-body pushing exercises include some form of elbow extension (straightening of the elbow joint).

In the early season it is common to experience fatigue, especially after long rides. This fatigue usually shows up in the hands, triceps (backs of the upper arms), trapezius muscles (upper back), and neck muscles.

These exercises may not help you ride any faster, but they will help develop balance between your upper body and lower body that can make cycling easier. Increased upper-body strength is particularly important to those specializing in mountain-bike riding.

Recommended upper-body pushing exercises include:

Bench Press: Lie on a flat bench with the barbell positioned above you. Grasp the bar with your hands shoulder-width apart. Lower the barbell to the center of your chest and raise it back to the starting position in a smooth, controlled motion. Do not arch your back or bounce the bar off your chest. Keep both feet planted on the floor. You may also perform this exercise using dumbbells.

Triceps Press (extension): This exercise can be done with a variety of implements attached to a high cable-pull apparatus. With palms facing down, grasp the handles and pull down, pinning your elbows at your sides. Hinging only at the elbows, lower the weight to a straight-arm position, then slowly return back to your starting point.

Overhead (shoulder/military) Press: Sit on an adjustable bench or upright chair positioned at 90 degrees with your back pressed firmly against the back-rest and your feet planted on the floor. With a shoulder-width grip on the bar, press the weight overhead. Slowly lower the weight to the top of the chest and press it back to the upright position.

UPPER-BODY PULLING EXERCISES Upper-body pulling exercises involve some form of elbow flexion (bending of the elbow joint). The upper body is particularly important because of its contribution to added strength and power when a cyclist is climbing hills or sprinting.

Recommended upper-body pulling exercises include:

Bent-Over Row: Place your palm and the same-side knee on a bench while keeping the opposite foot flat on the floor. Grasp a dumbbell with a palm-down grip on your open side. Keeping your back flat, pull the dumbbell up to the armpit, keeping the elbow pointed toward the ceiling. Lower the weight in a smooth, controlled motion. Place the opposite hand and knee on the bench and repeat with the other side. You may also perform this exercise with both arms simultaneously by using a barbell with a shoulder-width grip and pulling the bar to the center of the chest.

Arm (biceps) Curl: This exercise can be performed with a barbell, dumbbells, or a low-pull cable apparatus. Standing upright, grasp the barbell at shoulder width with your palms facing up. Curl the bar toward the chest, hinging at the elbows. Lower the weight to the starting position and repeat the movement.

Upright Row: Stand upright with your feet a few inches apart, and hold the barbell a few inches from the center with both hands, palms facing the body. Lift the barbell up toward the chin until it is at mid-chest height. The elbows should be pointing out. Hold the weight at the top of the movement for a count of two, and then lower it in a smooth, controlled motion.

LOWER-BACK EXERCISES Lower-back exercises are important because many cyclists experience back pain and fatigue, particularly early in the season or on long rides. While cyclists tend to be quite flexible in the area of trunk flexion (bending forward), they are notoriously poor at bending in the other direction (trunk extension). Training the lower-back muscles will help improve posture and will help transfer force to the pedals, especially when climbing in the saddle.

Recommended lower-back exercises include:

Back Extension: Using a back-extension bench (sometimes called a Roman chair), position yourself with your ankles locked behind the padded bars and your upper thighs resting on the padded platform. Your hips should be over the edge of the platform. With your arms across your chest, bend forward at the waist until the torso forms a 90-degree angle with the legs. Raise and lower yourself in a smooth, controlled motion. For added resistance, hold a weighted plate or ball across the chest.

Stiff-Legged Deadlift: (This is an advanced exercise; use extreme caution if you are inexperienced, or avoid it entirely.) Athletes who are highly flexible will need to elevate themselves on a sturdy platform or bench to reach full extension at the bottom of the movement. Stand on the elevated platform holding a barbell with a shoulder-width palms-down grip. Hinging only at the waist, lower the bar until you have reached full extension. You will feel the hamstrings tighten at the bottom of the movement. Rise back to the starting position in a smooth, controlled fashion, squaring your shoulders at the top of the lift.

ABDOMINAL EXERCISES The abdominal region is one of the weakest areas for many cyclists, and it needs to be one of the strongest. Your torso is the link between your upper body and your legs, and it needs to provide a stable platform for your legs to push against. If you have weak abdominal muscles, you won't be able to keep your torso and lower back stable when you push down on the pedals. Not only does this affect the power you can put into the pedals when sprinting and climbing, any weakness here can contribute to lower-back pain.

Recommended abdominal muscles include:

Trunk Curls (Abdominal Crunches): Lie flat on the ground with the knees bent at a 45-degree angle and the arms crossed over the chest. Curl your upper torso toward your knees, contracting the abdominal muscles and raising the shoulders off the ground. Only the shoulders should lift, not the lower back. Hold the contraction for a moment and then lower to the starting position. You should implement a variety of abdominal crunches that will work the upper, lower, and oblique muscles of the abdomen.

Sit-ups: Lie flat on the ground with the knees bent at a 45-degree angle and the hands interlocked behind the head. Rise up diagonally by hinging at the waist, keeping the elbows back. The chest should come close to touching the thighs at the top of the movement. Lower yourself back to the starting position. For advanced athletes, only lower the torso until the shoulder blades are two to three inches from the ground. For added resistance, hold a small weight plate or weighted ball behind the head or across the chest.

LOWER-BODY EXERCISES Most cyclists tend to overemphasize the lower body when strength training. In some instances this is an error, as more upper-body strength may be needed in order to obtain stability on the bike. The pedal stroke is a combination of hip-flexion and -extension and knee-flexion and -extension. The lower leg (calf) is not thought to contribute greatly to the pedal stroke, but some work should be directed here. I feel strongly that it's important to maintain the *same* range of motion when lifting as when cycling. This is why I don't prescribe weight training that includes a range of motion greater than your personal cycling motion.

Recommended lower-body exercises include:

Squat: While the squat can be considered the cornerstone of a cyclist's strength program, it is an advanced movement that requires excellent form and the use of a spotter. Athletes new to the gym should get proper instruction before attempting the movement. An Olympic safety cage is also recommended.

Place the barbell across the top of the shoulder blades so that it is cradled by the trapezius muscles. Beginners may want to pad the bar. Stand tall with the feet positioned at shoulder-width and the toes pointed slightly out. Lower the weight by bending at the knees. Keep the shoulders pulled back and do not round the back as you lower the weight. Cyclists only need to lower themselves to a knee-bend of 80 degrees, as this will closely approximate the knee angle at the top of a pedal stroke. Rise back to the starting position. Err on the conservative side with weight prescription so your form does not deteriorate.

Leg Press: Sit in a leg-press machine with the feet on the footplates in a shoulder-width stance. Upon releasing the safety latch, lower the weight by bending at the knees, forming a 90-degree angle with the upper and lower leg. Raise the weight in a smooth, controlled motion. Keep a slight bend in the knees at the top of the movement.

Leg Curl: Using a leg-curl machine, hook the ankles behind the lifting pads with the knees just over the bench's edge. Pull both heels toward the gluteus muscles as far as the machine will allow. Lower the weight in a smooth, controlled motion.

Calf (heel) Raise: This exercise can be performed on a seated calf-raise apparatus, leg-curl platform, or as a standing calf raise. After selecting the appropriate load, place the balls of the feet on the edge of the platform. Raise the weight by attempting to stand on the balls of the feet. Lower the weight by dropping the heels below parallel with the platform. Raise and lower in a smooth, controlled fashion.

Exercise Order

Once you have decided on the specific exercises, you need to determine the most effective order for performing them. I recommend that you first perform those exercises that use more than one body joint (multiple-joint movements). Single-joint movements, especially for the arms, are kept for the end of the workout. Training small muscles and single joints first will cause fatigue that can interfere with the proper performance of the more complicated, multiple-joint movements in which you will handle more weight. Use only multiple-joint movements during the Strength Phase. You will be handling heavier loads or performing quick movements, and performing these with only one joint could lead to injury. Also, as a cyclist, it may be best for you to exercise the lower body when you are most fresh, then move on to the upper-body exercises.

TRAINING INDOORS

Occasionally, you will be forced to perform your cycling workouts on a stationary trainer, and there are also certain ways indoor workouts can be more beneficial than outdoor training, such as:

- To create a controlled environment for environmental training (acclimatization, usually seen when training for events taking place in hot and humid locales)

- To enhance the ability to focus specifically on your workout
- To build the ability to ride continuously, without worrying about terrain, traffic, or weather
- To remove the limitations and negative dynamics of group rides/ training partners.
- To maximize the use of your limited time
- To create an ideal environment for performing technique exercises, such as FastPedal exercises
- To create an ideal environment to apply information learned from instructional videos

For the vast majority of athletes, I recommend limiting your indoor training sessions to a maximum of 2.5 hours. And when converting any outdoor training ride to an indoor workout, reduce the total ride length by 20 percent [see table below]. For rides of equal duration, you will generally expend more energy on an indoor trainer, compared with outdoors, due to the lack of stop signs, traffic lights, and descents. Your primary focus indoors should be to complete your specific workout tasks, rather than to complete the total workout time. In other words, after a thorough warmup, complete your specific tasks, such as FastPedal or SteadyState Intervals, and then complete any remainder of volume in ei-

Conversion of Outdoor to Indoor Ride Time

OUTDOOR TIME	INDOOR TIME (APPROXIMATE)
2.5 hours	2 hours
2 hours	1.5 hours
1.5 hours	1.25 hours
1 hour	45 minutes

ther an FM or an EM capacity as your time/comfort/patience allows, up to a total indoor-ride time of 2.5 hours.

Simulating your climbing position indoors is very useful for helping you develop good climbing technique regardless of where you live. Climbing changes your body position on the bike and increases the amount of muscle you are using, leading to an increase in heart rate at a given intensity level. By elevating your front wheel two to four inches above horizontal for workouts like MuscleTension Intervals and ClimbingRepeats, you can simulate your climbing position indoors. This is also very useful for athletes living in flat areas, like Miami, Florida, where I grew up.

While most workouts can be very effectively performed indoors, some don't make the transition very well. Examples include PowerStart, Stomps, and HighSpeedSprints. These are not very effective on an indoor trainer because the wheel can slip, and also because you're likely to spin out the resistance too quickly, unless you use a progressive resistance training.

When you move your training indoors, the risks of overheating and dehydration increase significantly. It is important to keep air moving around you so your sweat evaporates and cools your body the same way it does outdoors. With inadequate airflow, the air immediately surrounding your body heats up and gets extremely humid, but doesn't move. You become trapped in a "bubble" of hot, humid air that hinders your performance and increases your risk of heat stress. To minimize this risk, use one or more large fans to circulate the air. Also, consider lowering

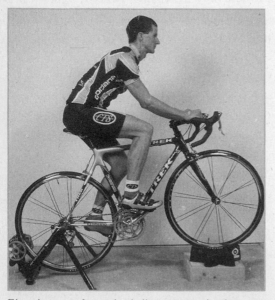

Elevating your front wheel allows you to simulate your climbing position while training indoors. *Photo © by Charlie Lengal III*

the thermostat or opening a window slightly to lower the temperature of your workout environment.

Even with fans blowing on you, your body tends to work harder to keep cool when you are training indoors. You need to drink more to minimize the effect of increased fluid loss that occurs through increased sweating. A good rule of thumb is to drink at least 50 percent more than you normally do while training outdoors. This is important, because as little as 2 percent body-weight loss due to dehydration can diminish performance. For example, if you weighed 150 pounds before a workout and 147 pounds after a workout, you lost 2 percent of your body weight due to dehydration, and most likely your performance suffered as a result. For every pound of body weight lost during a training session, you should take in 16 to 24 ounces of fluid soon afterward. Your goal, however, is to minimize the difference between your pre- and post-workout weights by drinking sufficient amounts of water and sports drinks.

Indoor Trainers and Spinning®

A stationary trainer is an essential piece of training equipment for every cyclist. If you need to purchase one, there are two basic types: resistance trainers and rollers. Resistance trainers usually include a device that rests against the rear wheel to create the resistance; the most common types are magnetic, wind, fluid, and electronic. I recommend a trainer that provides progressive resistance, as opposed to static resistance. Wind and fluid resistance units provide progressive resistance, which means that the resistance increases as your rear wheel moves faster, due either to a faster cadence or harder gearing. Static resistance, which is featured in magnetic resistance units, provides the same resistance regardless of your gearing or cadence, meaning you can effectively reduce the resistance you feel by increasing your cadence. Progressive resistance best simulates actual outdoor riding conditions.

Riding on rollers—a device on which you place your bicycle and ride it while balancing, as you would outdoors—is very useful for developing skill and technique because you have to balance atop three spinning rollers, but the required concentration often hinders your ability to perform specific workouts. If you purchase rollers that allow for added resistance, and you can ride rollers proficiently, you can perform FastPedal,

Tempo, and SteadyState workouts quite well. You can also complete FoundationMiles, EnduranceMiles, and RecoveryRides on rollers.

If you don't want to invest in a stationary trainer just yet, another alternative that you should consider is a "spinning" class. These have become quite popular in recent years, and should be available at various times at many of your local health clubs and fitness centers. Before you commit to a spinning class, make sure you confirm the instructor has a cycling background and is leading a cycling-based spinning class. What is a cycling-based spinning class? One that trains the energy systems in a progressive fashion, and that also mimics the types of efforts you may encounter in a typical group ride or a race. When deciding how many spinning classes to participate in, consider the intensity of the class. Some classes are very difficult, and you may spend a considerable portion of the time well above your lactate threshold. During the Foundation Period, which usually coincides with cold winter months, more than one hard spinning class per week can be detrimental to your overall training.

In November 2002, the CTS coaches and I launched a new kind of indoor training class in the CTS corporate offices in Colorado Springs, Colorado. Graber Products, Inc., supplied PowerTap™ powermeters to everyone enrolled in the class, and we used the CTS Field Test to establish power and heart-rate intensity ranges for each individual. From that session on, each individual in the class could work out with the support and camaraderie that make group training so enjoyable, and with individualized and precise training intensities that enhance the effectiveness of the training. People loved the classes, and the data we collected from the powermeters allowed us to immediately adjust workouts and intensity levels for each person in response to progress.

THE NEXT TOOL IN ENDURANCE TRAINING: ALTITUDE TRAINING TO IMPROVE PERFORMANCE

Numerous studies exist documenting the effects of altitude on physiological processes [see table on next page]. Atmospheric pressure is lower at altitude than at sea level, and because of this, when an individual temporarily goes to altitudes near 5,000 feet, the cardiovascular system has to work harder to keep blood-oxygen levels within normal ranges. Ventilation increases, as do resting HR and exercise HR. These changes are most noticeable in the first week at altitude, and they are more pronounced with greater changes in elevation. The numerous records set at the 1968 Olympics in Mexico City (elevation 7,300 feet) sparked an intentional effort by sports scientists and coaches alike to determine the process and benefits of altitude training for improved performance both at altitude and at sea level.

Physiological Benefits from Living at Altitude	
Increased ventilatory efficiency	Lungs have improved gas exchange ability
Increased total blood volume	Higher volume means distribution of oxygen-carrying red blood cells occurs more efficiently
Increased hematocrit levels	Represents an increased concentration of red blood cells in the total blood volume; more red blood cells means higher oxygen-carrying capacity

Until recently, most athletes who didn't live at altitude couldn't take advantage of these well-documented benefits because of the logistical complexities and costs associated with relocating to altitude. These athletes were always at a disadvantage both when traveling to altitude for competitions and when competing against those athletes who had the good fortune to be able to live at altitude. Even relocating temporarily (for as little as three to four weeks) to altitude to prepare for an important event is beyond the ability of most athletes.

To the benefit of all endurance athletes, two significant developments took place in the 1990s. The first was a groundbreaking study, published in the *Journal of Applied Physiology* (Levine and Stray-Gundersen, 1997) that demonstrated that a process for "living high and training low" improved athletic performance. About the same time, technological developments were being made in creating cost-effective artificial environments that could safely and accurately replicate altitude training at any elevation. Now there are commercially available artificial-environmental systems, such as those made by Colorado Altitude Training, in both room and tent formats. These allow the athlete to sleep at various altitudes ("live high") while having the ability to conveniently train in his or her local environment ("train low").

The most common possibilities for altitude vs. sea-level racing or training for most athletes include:

1. Living at sea level and competing at altitude. Racing at altitude when you live at sea level presents numerous physiological challenges. So, unless you have the ability to purchase a room or tent system a number of weeks (or preferably, months) before your competition, I recommend the following options:

   Best: Arrive at altitude at least three weeks (preferably four to six) prior to your competition for full acclimatization. You will need to reduce your training intensity and/or volume by 20 to 30 percent initially, and then gradually increase back to sea-level doses over the next two weeks.

   Good: Arrive at altitude at least two weeks before your competition. Reduce your training intensity and/or volume by 30 to 40 percent initially, and then gradually increase back to 75 to 85 percent of sea-level doses over the next ten days.

   Acceptable: Arrive at altitude within 24 hours of the scheduled competition, well rested and well hydrated. Though there is no scientific evidence that this is any more beneficial than arriving a few days before competition, I have found that athletes I've worked with competed best within one day of traveling to altitude. Reasons may include that they competed before dehydration or trouble sleeping affected their ability to perform.

2. Living at sea level and competing at sea level. By far the most common scenario for many athletes, competing at sea level pre-

sents no unique physiological challenges per se. However, appropriately utilizing the technologies of an artificial altitude environment, you can enhance your performance capabilities for sea-level competitions.

3. Living at altitude and competing at altitude. There are additional benefits to long-term exposure to altitude, in addition to those listed in Table on page 135, that further facilitate the body's ability to deal with a reduced atmospheric pressure. Elite athletes who live at altitude are now utilizing the artificial-environment technologies to further exploit the "live high, train low" concept. In a sense, they are "living high, training not-so-high." For example, if an athlete lives at 6,000 feet, she will set her room up to simulate an altitude of 9,000 feet.

4. Living at altitude and competing at sea level. Athletes who live at altitude and compete at sea level are at a measurable advantage compared to their sea-level counterparts. Athletes who live at altitude can also employ the artificial-environment technologies to again further exploit the "live high, train low" concept. For example, if an athlete lives at 6,000 feet, he will also have his room set up to simulate an altitude of 9,000 feet. Thus, he is "living" at 9,000 feet, "training" at 6,000 feet, and competing at sea level.

Making effective use of an artificial-altitude device can be complicated, and I recommend using one only in conjunction with working with a coach. There is a trade-off between the benefits of spending time in simulated altitude, and the possible detriments to your ability to recover. Some people have trouble getting quality sleep in an altitude tent or room, and you have to carefully consider the ways that poor sleep quality affects your workouts. There are also protocols related to the timing of when you sleep at altitude, especially in regard to the type of training you are doing. Those protocols are beyond the scope of this book, but it should be noted that, as with any training tool, correct use is the key to producing significant positive results. However, I will say that no technology, regardless of how sophisticated or effective, can make up for a poorly trained engine. So, make an effective training plan your first priority, and use the latest and greatest bells and whistles only to enhance adaptations you have worked so hard to achieve.

TRAINING BLOCKS

As this book progresses, you will find blocks of training at the ends of chapters (as well as menu plans at the end of Chapter 7). These training blocks are meant to guide you as you build your own yearly program, utilizing the information in the chapters and examples from real training plans.

Some people have the available time to train six days of the week; many more are restricted to four or five days. Many experienced racers, who have a great number of competitive seasons behind them, want to remain competitive but cannot devote as much time to training as they could when they were younger. With good planning and commitment, an athlete training four days per week can compete and do well in the amateur and Masters divisions in the United States. With people's time constraints in mind, I have provided training-plan examples for both six and five days per week. To adapt the five-day schedule to a four-day schedule, simply remove the Wednesday workout. If that still doesn't accommodate your work or family schedule, you can move the workout days around a little. Try to maintain one day between weekday workouts if you have back-to-back workouts on the weekend.

I have also broken the plans into Intermediate and Advanced categories. To determine which category you fall into, perform the CTS Field Test. Afterward, use the following table to determine your category:

INTERMEDIATE	ADVANCED
• Complete a 3-mile field-test effort in more than 8 minutes	• Complete a 3-mile field-test effort in less than 8 minutes
• Less than three years racing	• More than three years racing
• Struggle to finish hard local group rides with the "fast riders"	• Consider yourself one of the "fast riders" in your hard local group rides

Exactly as they are written, the training examples in this book may not perfectly match your schedule, current fitness level, and/or time availability. Consider your current number of weekly training hours before trying to implement any of the examples in this book. If you are currently training five hours per week, it is not a good idea to suddenly increase to eight or ten hours per week. Instead, reduce each day's proposed total workout time by 15-minute increments until the sum of weekly hours matches your availability and fitness level. Similarly, reduce the number of intervals if the training load in the example is significantly higher than what you are currently handling. Alternatively, reduce the frequency of interval workouts: i.e., two PowerStart workouts in a week instead of three. If you have to rearrange the workouts, use the following rule of thumb: alternate days of specific workouts (FastPedal, Tempo, SteadyState, etc.) with endurance or easy days during the week. It is all right to do two days of harder workouts back-to-back each week, and these usually fall on weekends.

Reading the Workouts

The workouts in this book are presented in the following manner:

2 hr FM w/4×3 min FP.

The translation for this notation is that you should ride for a total of two hours of FoundationMiles, and complete four FastPedal efforts of three minutes each within those two hours. The appropriate recovery times for individual workouts can be found in the workout descriptions section of Chapter 4.

Foundation Period Training Examples

	MONDAY	TUESDAY	WEDNESDAY	
Intermediate 5-Day				
Week 1	Rest Day	2hr FM w/5x10sec PS	1hr FM	
Week 2	Rest Day	2hr FM w/6x10sec PS	1.25hr FM	
Week 3	Rest Day	2hr FM w/7x10sec PS	1.5hr FM	
Week 4	Rest Day	1hr RR	1.5hr FM	
Advanced 5-Day				
Week 1	Rest Day	2hr FM w/7x10sec PS	1hr FM	
Week 2	Rest Day	2hr FM w/8x10sec PS	1.25hr FM	
Week 3	Rest Day	2hr FM w/10x10sec PS	2hr FM w/8x12sec S	
Week 4	Rest Day	1.5hr RR	2hr FM	
Intermediate 6-Day				
Week 1	Rest Day	2hr FM w/5x10sec PS	1hr FM	
Week 2	Rest Day	2hr FM w/6x10sec PS	1.25hr FM	
Week 3	Rest Day	2hr FM w/7x10sec PS	1.5hr FM	
Week 4	Rest Day	1hr RR	1.5hr FM	
Advanced 6-Day				
Week 1	Rest Day	2hr FM w/7x10sec PS	1hr FM	
Week 2	Rest Day	2hr FM w/8x10sec PS	1.25hr FM	
Week 3	Rest Day	2hr FM w/10x10sec PS	2hr FM w/8x12sec S	
Week 4	Rest Day	1.5hr RR	2hr FM	

	THURSDAY	FRIDAY	SATURDAY	SUNDAY
	2hr FM w/4x10sec PS	Rest Day	2.5hr FM w/30min RS	2hr FM w/3x3min FP
	2hr FM w/4x3min FP	Rest Day	2.75hr FM w/40min RS	2.25hr FM w/5x10sec PS
	2hr FM w/6x12sec S	Rest Day	3hr FM w/50min RS	2.5hr FM
	2hr FM w/5x12sec S	Rest Day	2.75hr FM w/45min RS	2hr FM w/5x12sec S
	2hr FM w/6x10sec PS	Rest Day	2.5hr FM w/45min RS	2hr FM w/3x5min FP
	2hr FM w/4x5min FP	Rest Day	2.75hr FM w/60min RS	2.25hr FM w/7x10sec PS
	1.5hr FM	Rest Day	3hr FM w/70 min RS	2.5hr FM
	2hr FM w/8x12sec S	Rest Day	2.75hr FM w/60min RS	2hr FM w/7x12sec S
	2hr FM w/4x10sec PS	45min RR	2.5hr FM w/30min RS	2hr FM w/3x3min FP
	2hr FM w/4x3min FP	1hr RR	2.75hr FM w/40min RS	2.25hr FM w/5x10sec PS
	2hr FM w/6x12sec S	1hr RR	3hr FM w/50min RS	2.5hr FM
	2hr FM w/5x12sec S	1hr RR	2.75hr FM w/45min RS	2hr FM w/5x12sec S
	2hr FM w/6x10sec PS	1hr RR	2.5hr FM w/45min RS	2hr FM w/3x5min FP
	2hr FM w/4x5min FP	1.25hr RR	2.75hr FM w/60min RS	2.25hr FM w/7x10sec PS
	1.5hr FM	1.25hr RR	3hr FM w/70 min RS	2.5hr FM
	2hr FM w/8x12sec S	1hr RR	2.75hr FM w/60min RS	2hr FM w/7x12sec S

6

Reinforcing Your Training Program

BEING A SUCCESSFUL CYCLIST means managing your energy. Everyone begins a race with a full tank of gas, and at the moment of truth the person with the most left in the tank has the greatest chance of winning. You work hard in training to develop energy systems and skills that give you power and speed. Don't put yourself at a disadvantage in races by burning energy unnecessarily. There are a lot of places where you can waste energy, and learning to conserve that energy and use it wisely is a large part of developing into a complete and successful competitor.

There are moments during every competition that determine your chances of winning. If you have the power and energy to initiate or respond to the right move, you can win the race. If you don't have the ability to recognize those moments, or can't put forth the effort required to take advantage of the opportunity presented to you, you have already lost the race.

Improving your riding technique improves your efficiency, which means that you have more energy available for the critical turning points of races. The way you pedal, the line you choose, and the position you hold in the peloton affect the amount of energy you use as you ride. Poor choices and poor riding techniques undermine the work you have done in training; the strongest rider in the race can often be defeated by smarter and more efficient racers.

THE ART OF GROUP RIDING

Groups rides are incredible tools that you can use to improve your racing performance, but many people misuse them to the point that they are detrimental to their overall training. Group rides offer several benefits to your training:

1. Increased motivation by training with partners
2. Increased ability to handle the energy demands of racing
3. Improved pack-handling skills
4. Increased comfort with high-speed riding

Group rides cannot take the place of specific workouts that address the development of your energy systems. They should be regarded as supplements to your training program and opportunities to add variety, racelike conditions, and tactical practice to your preparation for racing. Approach group rides like you would any other workout; establish goals for what you plan to accomplish during each group ride. These goals can range from learning to ride in close proximity to other riders, to spending a certain amount of time riding above your race intensity. Overreliance on group training undermines your aerobic development because of the inconsistent intensity that characterizes most group rides.

Using Group Rides to Improve Your Pack Skills

Drafting is your best way to conserve energy in races, and group rides are perfect places to learn how to stay out of the wind. Champions put their faces into the wind and force the pace, they don't follow wheels

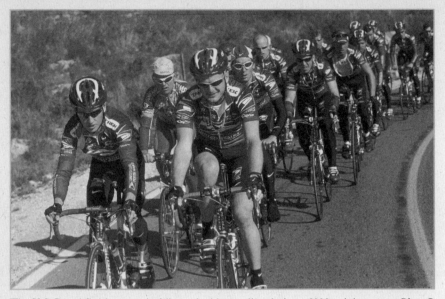

The U.S. Postal Service team is riding a double paceline during a 2002 training camp. *Photo © by Graham Watson*

all day and wait for the sprint. But they also understand that they will only have the power to attack the field or drive a breakaway if they hide in the shelter of the draft at all other times. Drafting is not an excuse to avoid doing your share of the work, it is a means of making the work you do more effective toward the goal of winning a race.

Most group rides operate on the principle of riding double-file, two-abreast, on the right side of the road. The first two riders pull the rest of the group through the wind, and their workload is about 30 percent higher than the load for the riders behind. When the riders up front decide to pull off, they each pull off to their respective sides and the rest of the group passes between them. They come back together at the back of the lines and ride in the draft until it is their turn to pull again. You can learn a lot just by riding in this type of formation.

It is important that you ride close together to get comfortable with riding in close proximity to other riders. When you are not comfortable with riders inches away from your handlebars, shoulders, and front wheel, you tend to grip the bars tightly and carry a lot of tension throughout your upper body. This is a waste of energy and a contributing factor in many crashes. You want to be relaxed, even if you overlap wheels with the rider ahead of you or bump into the rider next to you. Both of these things happen all the time in competition and you have to be used to dealing with them. Get used to running over potholes and obstacles instead of always dodging them. In races, you may not always have the luxury of moving around manhole covers and potholes. You should also practice eating and drinking in tight spaces, as you have to be able to maintain a straight line while doing so. An inexperienced rider may find it more comfortable to ride on the traffic (left) side of the group because he can maintain a comfortable distance from the rider to his right. He should work on gradually getting closer to that rider until he is riding shoulder-to-shoulder with him. An experienced rider should purposely ride on the gutter (right) side of the group so he has more space constraints to deal with. He has to maintain a tenuous position between the rider on his left shoulder and the edge of the road.

As the intensity of a group ride increases, the double-file style of riding often gives way to a single rotation paceline. In this formation, one line of riders advances (the advancing line) while the other falls back (the recovery line), and each rider takes an individual turn pulling at the front. You can usually maintain a higher overall speed with this type of paceline because the pulls are shorter and you can put out more power when you are at the front. Your individual speed and power output vary quickly as you ride in a rotating paceline. You have to increase your effort to maintain the group's speed as you get to the front and pull off. Do not, however, accelerate as you pull through. You goal is to maintain the group's speed, but in order to do that you will have to increase your effort level as you emerge from the draft. When you pull off, you have to decelerate slightly and drift back in the recovery line. When you reach the back, you have to judge when and how hard to accelerate to get back into the advancing line. If you accelerate too early or too hard, you will run up on the back of the rider ahead of you and have to tap your brakes. One tip for judging when to get ready to shift to the advancing line: remember the person who pulls off before you in the rotation. When you see that rider start to pass you, it is time to move over. Start moving over before he is completely past you so you can take full advantage of his draft. If he is already completely past you before you move over, you are

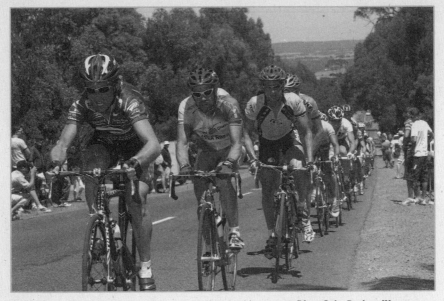

Single pacelines are more prevalent when the speed increases. *Photo © by Graham Watson*

out of his draft and will have to accelerate hard to get back into it. Again, you will most likely then have to tap the brakes to avoid running into him. Anytime you have to accelerate hard and then hit the brakes in a paceline, you have wasted energy.

Pacelines exist to help riders share the work of pushing through air resistance, so wind direction affects the way the paceline operates. The advancing line of riders should pull off into the wind if it is coming from the side. For example, if there is a light wind from the right, the advancing line should be on the left side and pull off to the right. If you turn a corner and the wind direction switches, the direction of rotation should also switch.

An echelon is the most appropriate formation for riding through side-winds, but you have to be wary of cars and traffic laws. An echelon is basically a rotating paceline that spreads diagonally across the road instead of in two straight lines. When the wind is coming in from the right, you have to move up to the left hip of the rider ahead of you in order to get a draft. Since the same is true for the riders behind you, every rider lines up on the hip of the next rider ahead. Like before, there is an advancing line and a recovery line, but this time the lines move diagonally across the road. Riding in a rotating echelon is an advanced skill, because you have to ride close together while being buffeted by side-winds. Your effort level changes frequently, and you have to be very comfortable with your handling skills in close spaces. The width of the road limits the number of riders who can be in an echelon, and this becomes a serious issue in racing situations.

In windy races like the spring classics in northern Europe, the peloton breaks up into several echelons because the roads are narrow. Riders fight to get into the first echelon, because they know that is where the strongest riders are. As soon as echelons form, the first echelon starts to pull away from those behind it. It is extremely difficult for a single rider to bridge the gap between echelons, and it is often fruitless anyway, because there is no room for him in the front echelon. It is very important to stay at the front of the peloton on windy days so you can get into the first echelon when it forms. If you find yourself too far back to make the first

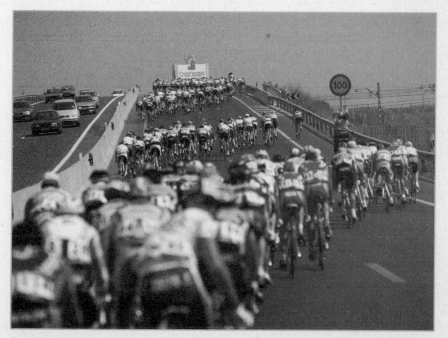

Strong winds from the right force the peloton into several echelons. Riding near the front of the peloton helps you get into the first echelon, where the strongest riders are. *Photo © by Graham Watson*

echelon, do not waste your energy fighting in the gutter for a nonexistent draft. Form a second echelon immediately. One of the biggest mistakes I see in amateur racing is the delay in establishing second, third, and fourth echelons. The longer you wait, the more energy you waste and the less chance you have of ever seeing the front of the race again.

Watch out for changes in the width of the road when riding in an echelon. If the road suddenly narrows, the riders who just moved from the recovery line to the advancing line will either ride off the road or find themselves in the gutter without a draft. Look ahead and anticipate narrowing roads. You may have to split the echelon or attack to the front of it and let the other riders fight for position in the back.

Using Group Rides to Improve Your Race-Fitness

Participating in group rides is a great way to fit some race-intensity rides into your training plan, and there are some specific ways you can make them effective tools for gaining race-fitness. The pace of group rides is often higher than the speed you could average on your own. This in itself is a benefit, because it teaches you to get accustomed to riding at high speed. Everything happens more quickly at high speed, and your reaction time quickens when you participate in group rides. You can also use a group ride to work on your cadence. Spin a lighter gear in high-speed groups so you learn to race with a high cadence.

You should generally do your share of work during a group ride, but sometimes it is good to utilize a group to help you complete interval work. Tell the other members of the group what you are planning to do beforehand so you don't aggravate them, and then start accelerating off the front for periods of one to three minutes. Between these intervals, get back into the group and stay in the draft to recover. Since the group's speed is high, you will be training yourself to recover while still riding fast. This is an essential skill for bridging the gap to breakaways or staying with the lead group after they chase down one of your attacks.

Training criteriums offer another opportunity to gain racing skills, because they feature an unstructured pack instead of an organized paceline. Successful racers find their way from the back of the peloton to the front without ever sticking their noses into the wind. You want to move up through the field instead of trying to accelerate around the outside of it. As a skill drill during training criteriums, start at the back of the group and try to move up to the front within one lap. Then return to the back of the group and do it again. In order to accomplish this, you have to be able to find or create openings between riders.

Learn to find spaces you can accelerate through. Look for diagonal lines, as these are less likely to close up on you. It is more difficult to move up between two riders whose handlebars are next to each other, because when they sense you between them, they will purposely stay close together to prevent you from moving up. You risk getting stuck between them with your bars dangerously close to two sets of whirring legs. Moving diagonally between riders is easier, because once you get your handlebars in front of someone else's, you can control where that rider goes.

To move diagonally between riders, you have to get your handlebars in front of the bars of the rider next to you. This allows you to deal one at a time with the two riders who border the space you are moving through. To move abreast of the rider ahead of you, you may need to create space by moving the rider next to you over. Since your bars are ahead of his, simply moving toward him forces him to either move over, tap the brakes, or accelerate in order to avoid hitting your legs with his handlebars. You should never have to take your hands off the handlebars to move through the peloton. You can use your shoulders and arms to protect your space and convince riders to let you move where you want to go, but using your hands to move a person over is dangerous and reveals deficiencies in your pack-riding skills. The only time it is acceptable to put a hand on a rider's shoulder or hip is to prevent a crash.

Training criteriums are also a good place to practice sprinting and attacking. One way to do this is to run the criterium similarly to a points race on the velodrome. You can establish that there will be a sprint every third or fourth lap of the criterium, and tactically prepare for each as if it were a finishing sprint. This allows you and others in the training race to experiment with different sprinting tactics. Try leading out the sprint one time and coming off wheels the next time. See what happens when you take inside and outside lines through the final corner. There are many ways to win bike races, and trying new tactics and maneuvers in training teaches you how to handle similar situations in competition.

Breaking Into the Line

TACTIC TIP: How many times has the field strung out into a single line and left you out in the wind trying to find a draft? You have two choices: go all the way to the back, or break into the line. Going to the back is not really an option. Riders are back there because they are having trouble keeping up, so getting behind them is not smart. When they get dropped, so will you. You have to break into the line, and no one is going to voluntarily let you in. Accelerate so you are shoulder-to-shoulder with a rider in the line. Start to drift back, and as soon as your handlebars clear his hips move over close to his rear wheel. Stay as close as possible to his rear wheel, and continue to drift back. This is kind of like backing into a parking space. The rider behind you won't be able stop you, because as you drift back and to the side, he has to either move over or back off before your rear wheel hits his front wheel. Most times you won't incur any wrath unless you break into the line and then proceed to let a gap open in front of you. That's why you want to get out of the wind as soon as possible, before you are so exhausted that even a draft won't help you.

HANDLING SKILLS: YOUR BIKE AS AN EXTENSION OF YOUR BODY

It can be difficult for experienced racers to describe accurately how they corner or climb or sprint. Their level of experience and skill makes their actions second nature, so fluid that they no longer have to consciously think about them. The bicycle becomes an extension of the body, and you develop an amazing agility and feel for the road. Getting to this level of technical skill is important, because it frees you to concentrate on winning races instead of just surviving them. The goals of technical skills are increased safety and efficiency. A technically proficient rider conserves energy by minimizing the energy he uses between the start and finish of a race.

Cornering

You have to be nimble on your bike to dive through corners quickly and safely. You need to be able to move your bike under you as you shift your weight and change direction. There are two main tenets of cornering: planting your weight on your outside pedal, and leaning the bike instead of your body. Both of these things work together to keep your center of gravity over your tires so you maintain traction. You can slide out in a perfectly smooth, dry turn if you lean over too far, because the farther you lean your body into a corner, the farther your center of gravity moves away from your tires.

Adjust your speed as you approach a corner, not while you are in the middle of it, and look through the turn instead of looking at it. Looking through the turn helps keep your body upright and over the tires as you lean the bike over. If you have trouble tipping the bike into the turn, focus on pushing your handlebars into the inside of the corner; extend your inside arm. This works for criterium corners as well as turns on descents.

Improving your cornering skills helps you win races. In a typical four-corner criterium, you may turn as many as 400 times, so saving energy by cornering efficiently can make the difference between sprinting for the win and dropping off the back. Accelerating out of corners requires a lot of energy, and your goal is

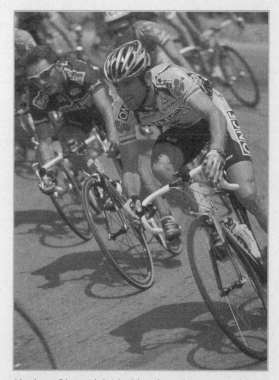

Abraham Olano (right) looking through a corner, with his weight on his outside foot. *Photo © by Graham Watson*

to maintain your momentum through corners so you don't have to accelerate as hard coming out.

Tight courses and the battle for position often lead to an accordion effect in corners. The front of the field gets through the corner quickly, but as riders start to slow down to negotiate the corner, the riders behind them have to slow down even more. The more you have to slow down going into a corner, the harder you have to accelerate coming out of it. The obvious way to avoid the accordion effect is to ride near the front of the peloton, but you also need to know what to do when you are in the rear 85 percent of the field.

The character of the racecourse affects the most efficient cornering lines in a criterium. Your goal is to maintain your speed so you can move up in the field through smart positioning instead of hard efforts. You may be able to conserve your speed on the outside of the turn, but then you risk getting shoved into the curb by the riders who took the inside line. If the field is coming to almost a complete stop in the inside of a turn, you may be able to ride around 30 racers by taking the outside line.

Climbing

Great climbers make ascending mountain peaks look easy, because their bodies are relaxed and they are not fighting against their bicycles. Their relaxed demeanor hides the fact that sustained climbing efforts are some of the most taxing on cyclists' energy systems. Relaxing your upper body on climbs, including the muscles of your neck, head, and face, saves important energy that your legs and lungs crave. Your aerobic and lactate-threshold training increases your power on climbs, but riding economically increases your speed.

Body Position   The most economical climbing position is seated with your hands on the tops of the handlebars. Since the saddle is supporting a lot of your body weight, your cardiovascular system does not have to supply oxygenated blood to as many working muscles as when you are standing on the pedals. Not only is your heart rate lower, but also you can breathe more easily because your upper body is not crunched up. As a result, you are increasing the amount of oxygen you are taking in while limiting the body's increase in demand for oxygen. You may find that it takes time before you can tolerate staying seated for long climbs, but the benefits are well worth the training required.

When you do have to stand up on climbs, it is usually to stretch or accelerate. In either case, shift into a higher gear before rising out of the saddle. When you stand up you can take advantage of your body weight as well as the power in your legs, meaning you can push a bigger gear. Your cadence will most likely decrease when you stand as well, so pushing a bigger gear is necessary for maintaining your

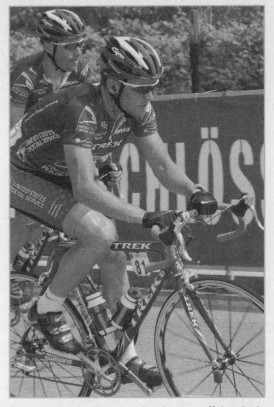

Lance Armstrong demonstrating the most efficient body position for climbing. *Photo © by Graham Watson*

speed. Be careful not to anger the rider behind you by shoving your bike back into him as you rise from the saddle. This happens when you pull back on the handlebars to lift yourself up over the bars. Instead, use your leg to lift your body (like you are climbing stairs) as it begins the downstroke. Your downstroke will be powerful because of your body weight, but there will be a lull in power when that leg hits the bottom of the stroke. This is what causes trouble for the rider behind you. To prevent a loss of momentum, slightly force your bike forward under you as your leg reaches the bottom of the pedal stroke. You'll give your second leg the split second it needs to cross the top of the pedal stroke without costing you your precious momentum. Saving forward momentum saves energy and keeps the rider behind you happy.

Pack Positioning Your pack position at the base of a climb can have a huge effect on your position at the summit. Start climbs near the front of the peloton whenever possible. First of all, the field often splits on climbs, and you don't have to catch back up to the front group if you are already in it. If you can't keep up with the leaders, starting climbs at the front of the peloton also allows you to slip back gradually through the field without dropping completely off the back. You may start the climb at the front and be passed by 150 riders, but getting to the summit with riders around you is always better than having to chase back on by yourself.

There is often a rubber-band effect over the top of climbs. The front of the field crosses the summit and starts descending. As the stretched-out field follows behind, each rider has to accelerate harder over the top in order to hold on to the wheel ahead of him. The leaders ride a sustainable pace over the summit, but the riders behind are forced into a maximal effort just to maintain contact. The irony of the situation is that the riders at the back are the ones struggling to keep up on the climb in the first place; and just based on their position, they have to hit the gas the hardest over the final 100 meters of the hill. Work harder to stay or move up in the field toward the top of climbs to avoid having to force the pace over the summit. The additional work during the climb will be less detrimental than the maximal effort necessary at the top.

Pedal Cadence Learn to pedal faster on climbs. A lot has been made of this since Lance started winning the Tour de France with a high climbing cadence. The technique works because it shifts some of the work of climbing from the leg muscles to the cardiovascular system. You can create 450 watts of power pedaling quickly or slowly, but the more quickly you pedal, the less force you have to exert during each pedal stroke. However, there is an energy cost to pedaling faster. Increasing your cadence burns a lot of oxygen because you have to contract all the muscles necessary for a pedal stroke more frequently. But because there is plenty of oxygen in the blood and the increased demand for oxygen is spread among many muscles, each can get the oxygen it needs for continued contractions without resorting to anaerobic metabolism. Producing the same amount of power with a lower cadence is problematic, because muscular fatigue sets in quickly as lactic acid builds up in leg muscles.

Skeletal muscle fatigues in a different manner than the cardiovascular system does, and given the choice between increasing the load on skeletal muscle or on the cardiovascular system, choose your heart and lungs over your legs. Breathing faster and raising your heart rate increase the amount of energy you burn, but with proper nutrition and hydration your cardiovascular system can support the increased load far longer than your leg muscles can. Staying aerobic longer means accumulating less lactic acid and sparing more muscle glycogen, both of which help you stay fresh for the end of the race and recover more quickly afterward.

Mastering Switchbacks The shortest distance between two points is not always the best route. How you climb through a switchback affects how much energy it costs you. The inside line is the shortest distance, but it is also the steepest pitch. The outside line is longer, but because it is shallower you can maintain your speed with less increase in your power output. Riding the steep inside line causes a surge in your power output; you are exerting a huge effort to save a few feet. You can maintain your climbing rhythm, and conserve or even gain speed, by climbing the outside line through a switchback.

On the other hand, you can take advantage of the steep inside line to attack the group. A hard acceleration anywhere on a climb costs a lot of energy, but you get the greatest benefit from your effort when you attack on steep pitches. You can quickly open up a large gap, and your rivals will have to dig deep to accelerate hard enough to catch you. This is another reason to climb with a high cadence. It is easier to accelerate when you are already pedaling fast. Remember Lance Armstrong's "look back" attack on Alpe d'Huez in the 2001 Tour de France? He attacked in the first few kilometers of the climb, because that is where the pitch is the steepest. Jan Ullrich was riding a bigger gear, with a lower cadence, and could not accelerate the gear as quickly as Lance could accelerate his. Lance had opened up a significant gap by the time Ullrich muscled the bigger gear up to speed. The gap remained almost the same all the way to the summit, illustrating that the two men were climbing at essentially the same speed. Lance won the stage because he was able to use the steepness of the pitch to his advantage and get away from his rival. You don't have to climb faster than everyone else; you just have to get away from everyone else and then settle back into a sustainable speed and rhythm.

Shift Up as You Approach the Summit Relief is in sight as you approach the top of a climb, but be careful not to relax too soon. When the slope begins to level off, the resistance against you lessens, and many riders welcome the opportunity to reduce their power output. The problem is, riders who continue working hard all the way over the climb gain precious time on you when you relax too early. To avoid this, shift into bigger gears and accelerate over the top of the climb. There will be plenty of time to recover on the descent, so consider the real top of the climb to be 50 meters after you start descending.

Descending

The best descenders are smarter, not necessarily more courageous. Safely maneuvering down a mountain at up to 60 mph is a matter of skill, and you don't have to be a daredevil to descend well. Relax and move smoothly over the bike. The more tightly you grasp the handlebars, the more skittish your steering becomes. Momentum is the key to maintaining high speed on descents. You don't want to hit the brakes any more than you absolutely have to, because it takes a long distance and a lot of work to regain the momentum you lose through braking. Correctly setting up for a high-speed corner is absolutely critical. You have to choose a good line, because you don't have time to adjust it once you commit to the path. Try to choose a line that passes through the apex of a tight turn, but don't cross the centerline of the road unless you are racing on closed roads. Start far out on the opposite side of the road; brake before the turn, look through it, lean the bike (keeping the body upright over the wheels) into the turn, and come out wide on the exit from the turn. Plant your weight on your outside foot. If the turn is off-camber (slanted toward the outside instead of banked to the inside of the turn), keep the bike more upright than normal to avoid sliding out. Descend with your hands on the drops of your bars to ensure that there is sufficient weight over the center of the bike. The bike should be doing all the leaning underneath you, to the point that it should be difficult for me to tell that you are turning at all if I am looking only at your body.

Everything happens faster when you are going downhill, and your reaction time has to adjust accordingly. Look far ahead for obstacles or upcoming corners because you don't have much time to prepare. If you are descending at 60 mph, you are covering 300 feet (the length of a football field) every 3.4 seconds. That's not much time to spot, recognize, and deal with rocks, gravel, or potholes in your path. Remember that slight handling adjustments are amplified at high speed. The faster you are going, the less drastic your movements should be.

Pedaling on descents helps blood continue to circulate rapidly through your legs, because muscle contraction speeds the venous return of blood back to the heart. Your body takes care of itself in terms of circulating blood to your muscles and organs, but after hard efforts, your circulation slows a little bit and blood pools in your lower limbs. That blood is not oxygenated and contains a lot of lactate, so your body wants to get it back to the heart and lungs as quickly as possible. Many times there are several hills or mountains in a row, and pedaling down the first descent makes the subsequent climbs a little easier. Your legs feel fresher because light to moderate pedaling downhill has helped clear out the lactic acid that accumulated during the climb. You don't get the heavy, sluggish sensation that occurs when you work hard up a climb, coast down the other side, and then try to ride hard again.

Professional cyclists are great descenders, but accidents still happen. Remember when Jan Ullrich misjudged a turn and flew off the road into a creek during the 2001 Tour de France? Johan Bruyneel, the U.S. Postal Service team's Director Sportif, knows all about that too. He missed a turn in the Alps and went flipping off the side of a steep embankment. I can't say I escaped descents unscathed either. I was once involved in a pileup while descending through a tunnel. I emerged from the tunnel with someone else's bike and only one shoe!

Sprinting

Good sprinters win bike races, but sprinting skills are also imperative for initiating and bridging to breakaways, accelerating out of corners,

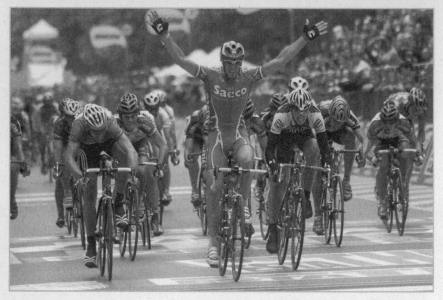

Great technique is as important as power and speed when it comes to winning sprint finishes.
Photo © by Graham Watson

and maintaining field position. Sprint training is beneficial because it reinforces good bike-handling skills while also improving your maximum power output. There are three parts to every sprint: the jump, the acceleration, and the top end.

The Jump Your initial jump is very short but extremely powerful. You're applying maximum power to the pedals in an attempt to accelerate fast enough to get away from the riders around you. A rider with a strong jump can open up a few bike-lengths on the field in the beginning of a sprint. If you can follow a strong jump with good acceleration and top-end speed, you have a good chance of winning the sprint. It's like getting a head start; everyone else has to catch up to you. Workouts like PowerStarts are great for developing the muscular power necessary for accelerating quickly.

The Acceleration Once you have initiated your sprint with the jump, you have to accelerate to maximum speed. It is tempting to immediately shift all the way to your biggest gear, but then your cadence would fall as

> **TACTIC TIP:** Jump in a smaller gear than you think you should. Just like when you attack on climbs, you can accelerate a smaller gear more quickly than you can a big one. Jump in a small gear to get the sprint going quickly, then start shifting up as you spin out the gear.

you struggle against the drastically increased resistance. Your shifting should be based on cadence, much the same way you use a tachometer in a stick-shift car. Get your leg speed (rpm) up before you shift so you don't bog down in the harder gear. For example, jump in a 53×17 and accelerate the gear to 130 rpm. When you shift to your 53×15, your cadence will drop due to increased resistance from the gear. If you were to skip the 15 and shift from the 17 to the 13 or 12, your cadence would fall even more because the increase in resistance is greater. Instead, accelerate the 53×15 up to 130 rpm before you shift to the 53×14 or 13. Then get *that* gear up to 130 rpm and shift again. By using more gears, you lessen each increase in resistance, and you accelerate like a rocket. SpeedAccelerations, FlatSprints, and HillSprints all develop the acceleration component of your sprint.

Top-End Speed Your jump and acceleration get you ahead of everyone else, and then you have to sustain that speed so they don't catch you. Ideally, you're still accelerating when you cross the finish line, but at the very least you don't want to be slowing down in the final 100 meters. Having great top-end speed means being able to sustain your maximum power for up to 20 seconds of an anaerobic effort. Many riders train the first two parts of their sprints and neglect top-end speed. They look great coming out of the last corner and fade as the entire field streams by them before the line. To train your top-end speed, use PowerIntervals and SpeedIntervals to improve your tolerance for lactic acid. Extended maximum efforts cause a great deal of lactic acid to accumulate in muscles, and your lactate tolerance partially determines how long you can maintain that intensity before having to slow down.

Different Sprints for Different People Cyclists come in all shapes and sizes and are better adapted to different types of sprints. Big, tall, powerful riders often have great top-end speed, but they need the sprint to start early because it takes longer for them to accelerate. Smaller riders often have better jumps because of their power-to-weight ratios, but they don't have the muscle mass to produce the maximum power needed for great top-end speed. Shorter sprints, especially those that start from lower speeds or just after a corner, and uphill sprints favor the smaller rider.

As a race enters the final ten kilometers, you should have an idea of how it is going to finish. As a smaller rider looking at a probable field sprint, attacking is probably your best strategy. Try to break up the field, or at least tire out the big sprinters by making them chase you. Repeated attacks near the end of a race cause confusion. Everyone looks at one another, waiting for someone else to chase. A slight hesitation in the field is all you need in order to get away and win.

Keeping the pace extremely high in the final ten kilometers tends to discourage attacks from smaller riders, making this the best strategy for more powerful sprinters. It is really hard to attack and stay away from a field that is already going 40 mph, and only riders who can produce massive power outputs can accelerate out of a draft at those speeds. Professional teams hire riders specifically to keep the pace high, because the speed effectively reduces the number of riders in contention for the win. Amateur racers rarely have the luxury of a team lead-out, and individual riders have to work together to make the situation work for them. If you desire a field sprint, take the initiative. Find the powerhouse riders in the field, go to the front, and drive the pace. In the end, several of you will sprint for the win without having to worry about the rest of the racers who are strung out halfway around the course. Depending on what kind of finish best suits you, take the race into your own hands. Be a factor in the finish and either take advantage of a situation that is good for you or recognize your disadvantage and seek to change the situation.

HANDLING ROAD CONDITIONS

Preparing for adverse conditions is part of training for competition. The weather won't always cooperate on race day, but a good racer knows how to adapt to poor conditions and, in some cases, take advantage of them.

Rain

Train outside on rainy days and get used to being soaked to the bone. I'm not saying you shouldn't use rain capes or waterproof shells, but I am saying that if you don't know what it's like to train hard when you're soaked and cold, you're going to have trouble if it starts raining during a road race. Rain negatively affects the way racers compete, because they associate wetness with misery. They're less aggressive and more likely to huddle together in a big group. Look at rainy races as opportunities. A breakaway is a safer place to be on wet roads anyway, and the field may be more willing than usual to let you go.

A few rainy-road tips:

1. Wet steel is slicker than a frozen pond. Riding straight over manhole covers or railroad tracks is fine, but avoid cornering over them if possible. The same holds true for painted lines and crosswalks. If you have to corner over lines or manhole covers, keep the bike more upright than you normally would. When you lean a bike, there is a force perpendicular to the road and another force parallel to the road. The farther you lean, the greater

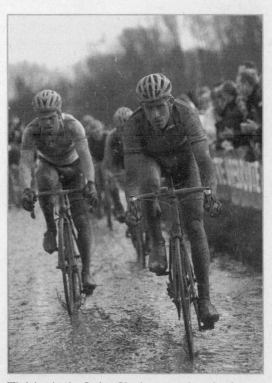

Thriving in the Spring Classics means knowing how to handle poor road and weather conditions. *Photo © by Graham Watson*

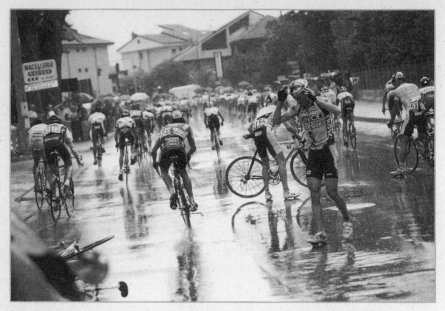

Rain can turn any road into a dangerously slick surface. *Photo © by Graham Watson*

the force parallel to the road. If the parallel force is less than the friction between your tire and the road, you stay up. If the force is greater than the friction, the wheel slides. Rain reduces the friction between your tires and the road, and keeping the bike more upright on slick surfaces reduces the force that is parallel to the road, meaning you are less likely to slide out in a corner if you keep your bike more upright.

2. Be wary of puddles. It's very hard to tell if there's a deep pothole in the center.

3. Your brakes barely work. Granted, technology has improved, and so has stopping power in wet conditions, but it still takes longer to stop in the rain. Plan ahead.

Sand/Gravel/Dirt

Treat sand and gravel much the same way you treat wet steel and road paint. Even in dry conditions, sand and gravel are slippery. Try to ride straight through them instead of cornering through them. If there is sand or gravel in a corner, keep the bike more upright than usual to avoid sliding out. Dirt, sand, and gravel aren't enemies for good road riders, though. I believe it is good to get your road bike dirty occasionally by taking it off the pavement.

Many of the skills that apply to road and criterium racing require good mobility and agility on your bike. Riding in the dirt is a great way of challenging your handling skills so you become even more confident in your ability to control your bike on the road. I grew up in Florida, and now I live in Colorado. Both places have plenty of pavement and endless miles of dirt roads. When you ride on dirt roads or paths, you get used to the feeling of being less solidly connected to the ground than you are when you ride on pavement. As you become more comfortable, you learn to handle bumps, small slides, and softer sand without thinking about it. This makes you more confident on the dirt, but more important, it elevates your overall feel for handling a bike to the point that you can stay upright through anything.

The CTS offices are in Colorado Springs, where the rocky and sandy soil moves under your feet. The coaches who live and work here have many ride routes that include extended stretches of dirt. One such route is in Cheyenne Canyon, a three-mile climb that rises more than 1,500 feet above the city. You can climb on pavement or on dirt, and I know several CTS employees who much prefer to descend on the dirt road. And after flying down the wide, sandy road, there's a choice. You can ride back to the city on pavement or take a shortcut down a curvy and loose singletrack trail. The singletrack is more fun and challenging, and as a result the bikes hanging in the office are often covered with a fine layer of red dirt. I've definitely noticed that several employees' handling skills have drastically improved. Find some tame dirt trails in your area—gravel bike paths work well for starters—and incorporate them into your training rides. Be careful not to get in over your head, though. Road bikes and road wheels are not designed for drop-offs, log crossings, etc.

CYCLING POSITION

The body is adaptable and the bicycle is adjustable, but there is much greater adjustability in the bicycle and its components than there is adaptability in the body. I abide by the concept of accommodative fitting for the bicycle: finding the optimum position of the body on the bicycle to meet your most common cycling goals. There are several effective formulas for deriving a good position on the bike, and I have found that they all provide a good starting point, but none is 100-percent accurate for all cyclists. Bicycle positioning, just like training, should be individualized. Cycling is a highly repetitive activity that creates opportunity for overuse injuries caused by problems with muscular strength, coordination, flexibility, or skeletal alignment. Precise fit must take those factors into consideration, as well as the relative strength of supporting muscles in the torso and the upper body. It is also important to consider your cycling goals as they relate to your positioning. If you are primarily participating in long, noncompetitive endurance events, your cycling position should focus on comfort over aerodynamics.

Remember that adapting to changes in bicycle position takes time, and that you should make changes only to fix problems. In many cases, the old adage "If it isn't broken, don't fix it" applies to bike fit.

The results of having good position on the bike should be obvious. A properly positioned rider:

- can ride comfortably with hands on the drops for extended periods of time while breathing normally.
- is not limited by pain or numbness in the neck, shoulders, hands, low back, or knees.
- can keep hips level while pedaling at most cadences.
- can handle a bicycle with confidence and minimize the potential for losing traction from the road.

Maneuvering your bicycle is easy when your bicycle fits you well. You can corner in or out of the saddle and sprint holding on to the brake hoods or the drops. If your bike is too big for you, or your position is too stretched-out, you may have difficulty maneuvering quickly; the bike may handle sluggishly and you may feel like you're driving a boat instead of a racing bike. On the other hand, riding too small a frame leads to the opposite effect: a small bike or a cramped position makes handling twitchy and nervous. Instead of handling the bike effortlessly, you have to ride carefully to maintain stability.

Your weight distribution between your front and back wheels can drastically affect the way your bike handles. Weight distribution is a function of where your three basic contact points (foot to pedal, buttocks to saddle, and hands to handlebar) are. Your head and shoulders are heavy and can significantly affect your weight distribution. Too little weight on the front end can lead your front wheel to slide out in a turn or cause the front end to wobble at high speeds. Changes in your reach to the handlebars (a.k.a. cockpit position) can affect handling. Variables include such things as close or distant proximity of the saddle to the bar, and excessive height or depth of the bar.

Common Fit-Related Pain Syndromes

There are several common bike-related pain syndromes, but diagnosing them is rarely simple. Pain syndromes often result from a combination of bike fit, musculoskeletal challenges, and training errors (too much too quickly). The table below lists the most common pain

Common Pain Syndromes and Their Pathomechanics

Anterior knee pain (front)

poor quadriceps flexibility	regular, proper stretching
poor cleat alignment	define and align cleat to neutral
low saddle position	increase saddle height to normal
forward saddle position	normalize to knee over pedal spindle
excessive quadriceps use in pedaling	increase cadence, use single-leg pedaling to help normalize pedaling
prolonged low cadence	increase cadence, use cadence monitor on bicycle computer for feedback
excessive crank length	shorten crank length to suggested

Common Pain Syndromes and Their Pathomechanics *(continued)*

Posterior knee pain (back of knee, hamstrings)

poor cleat alignment	define and align cleat to neutral
excessive saddle height	lower and normalize saddle height
saddle too far back	saddle forward, knee over pedal spindle
excessive cleat float	limit float to 6 degrees total (3 degrees side)

Lateral knee pain (outside, iliotibial band)

poor hamstring flexibility	regular, proper stretching
poor cleat alignment—toes point in	define and align cleat to neutral
extreme height of saddle	lower and normalize saddle height
low saddle height	raise and normalize saddle height
narrow stance-width on pedals	widen and normalize stance-width on pedals

Medial knee pain (inside)

weak lateral hip muscles	strengthen core and lateral hip musculature
poor cleat alignment—toes point out	define and align cleat to neutral
excessive stance-width on pedals	narrow and normalize stance-width on pedals

Neck and shoulder pain

improper tilt of saddle	normalize/neutralize saddle tilt
excessive reach to handlebar	lessen reach to bar via stem-length
limited reach to handlebar	increase reach to bar via stem-length
handlebar too low	raise the level of the handlebars

Common Pain Syndromes and Their Pathomechanics *(continued)*

Lower-back pain

poor hamstring flexibility	regular, proper stretching
poor gluteal flexibility	regular, proper stretching
excessive reach to handlebars	
reach	lessen reach to bar via stem-length
depth	raise the level of the handlebars
improper tilt of saddle	normalize/neutralize saddle tilt
degenerative changes in spine	refer to healthcare provider
poor core strength	stomach/back strength
	stomach/back coordination

Numb/painful hands

low saddle tilt	normalize/neutralize saddle tilt
improper reach to bars	
too long	lessen reach to bar via stem-length
too short	increase reach to bar via stem-length
improper padding	better bar tape (cork)
	increase overlap of tape
	well-padded gloves
single hand position on handlebar	frequent change of hand position on handlebars

Numb/painful feet

forward cleat position	cleat under ball of foot
mechanical dysfunction of foot	orthotic from qualified healthcare provider
shoe too small	normalize shoe size
excessive quadriceps use in pedaling	increase cadence, use single-leg pedaling to help normalize pedaling
prolonged low cadence	increase cadence, use cadence monitor on bicycle computer for feedback

syndromes and their possible pathomechanics. This is intended to give you a starting point to investigate some of your own bike-fit issues, but it is not intended to diagnose or cure problems. One of the coaches I work with closely has spent a great deal of time examining the marriage of athlete and bicycle. Erik Moen is the CTS Director of Health Services, a physical therapist, and a certified strength and conditioning specialist who has been performing professional bike-fit services for clients for more than ten years. Both he and I suggest that you consult a qualified professional to assist in diagnosis and treatment of bike-related pain syndromes.

Asymmetrical lower-extremity pain may suggest asymmetry of muscular development, fit asymmetry, or bony asymmetry.

Getting Started with a Self-Fit

The basic fitting of your bicycle requires a stationary trainer, your bicycle, appropriate bicycle tools, a plumb bob, and a mirror. Ensure that your bicycle is level by using a bubble level on the top-tube. For sloping top-tubes, measure the height of the hubs from the ground.

Critical Bike Measurements

Always take measurements of your bicycle prior to making any adjustments, so you can reverse them if you need to. You should also get into the habit of marking some parts of your bike, like the seatpost and seat rails, so you can quickly reset them if they get moved. Record the measurements in your training log, because you never know when you may need them. On U.S. National Team trips, it was not uncommon for bored racers to take a coach's or other rider's bike completely apart, as a joke.

Fitting the Endurance Cyclist

As a serious cyclist, you spend an enormous amount of time on your bike, so it makes sense to ensure that you are comfortable in a position in which you may spend three, four, or maybe many more hours at a time. Bike fit focuses on your three contact points with the bicycle: pedals, seat, and handlebars, in that order. Below are the steps that Erik Moen uses to measure and adjust a cyclist's riding position, listed in order from the first task to the last.

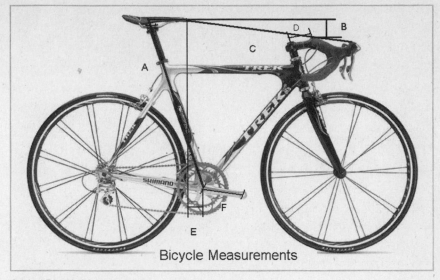

Bicycle Measurements

Critical Bicycle Measurements.
A= Seat height: Middle of bottom bracket to top of saddle
B=Vertical difference bewtween saddle and top of bars
C=Ultimate reach: Tip of saddle to tip of brakehood
D=Length of stem
E=Seat set back: horizontal difference between tip of saddle and bottom bracket
F=Crank length

1. Establish Cleat Position

For your records: Record your pedal style, cleat style, and the amount of cleat rotation allowed. Cleat position is easily marked by tracing with a permanent marker. Stack height is defined as the distance from the center of the pedal spindle to the bottom of the shoe. Different shoe/cleat/pedal combinations have various total heights, depending on the thickness of the shoe sole, the thickness of the cleat, and the manner in which the cleat secures to the pedal. When you change pedal systems or shoes, you have to be careful to consider how a possible change in stack height or sole thickness can affect your saddle height.

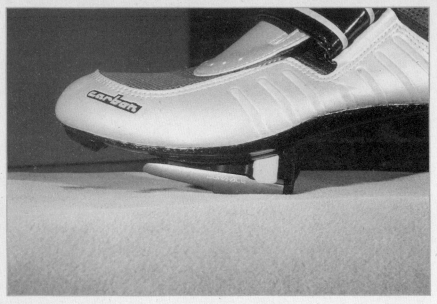

Stack height of pedal/cleat/shoe. *Photo © by Charlie Lengal III*

Adjusting Cleat Position: In general, the ball of the foot should be centered over the pedal spindle, which means that the head of the third metatarsal bone should be directly above the spindle. The third metatarsal head is located at the base of your third toe (the metatarsal at the base of the big toe is the first metatarsal). This accomplishes effective leverage to the pedal combined with greater potential for foot comfort with endurance pedaling. A suggested cleat placement is frequently in line with the first metatarsal head. This position is slightly forward of our suggested position.

Besides the fore/aft position of the foot, you also need to look at its lateral rotation. Most modern clipless pedals allow for varying amounts of float, but signs that your cleats are not properly aligned include: difficulty getting the cleat in or out of the pedal; irregular pain at the ankle, knee, or hip; and premature release of the cleat in situations under load (such as a sprint or when executing a track-stand).

2. Shoe Inserts

Shoe inserts are generally advised to enhance foot comfort. Common off-the-shelf shoe inserts are designed to be accommodative support of the foot. Custom orthotics and shims can be useful when treating foot dysfunction or skeletal problems. Before using either custom orthotics or shims, consult a physician or qualified practitioner to make sure you need them.

3. Saddle Height

For your records: Measure from the middle of the bottom bracket along the seat-tube/post to the top of the saddle. Mark the seat-post at the level of the top of the seat-tube.

Adjusting Saddle Height: The best method for determining proper saddle height is measuring the angle of your knee when the pedal is at dead bottom center (DBC). At DBC, the crank is in line with the seat tube of the bicycle, not pointed straight at the ground. This represents the longest distance between the saddle and the pedal. The typical knee-flexion angle established for the endurance road cyclist is 25 to 35 degrees and is measured using a goniometer. A good starting angle is 32 degrees. Care should be taken to ensure that your foot is in the position it would be in while pedaling at or around 90 rpm. Avoid the temptation to drop your heel when you reach DBC, as this will skew your measurement. People with posterior knee pain, poor hamstring flexibility, or lower-back pain may need to maintain a lower saddle position (knee angle greater than 32 degrees). A higher saddle position (knee angle less than 32 degrees) is suitable only for those with good flexibility.

There are a few other methods of determining saddle height. Greg LeMond first published one method that is widely used. This method calculates saddle height by multiplying your inseam length by 0.883. This gives you a measure from the center of the bottom bracket to the top of the saddle, along the length

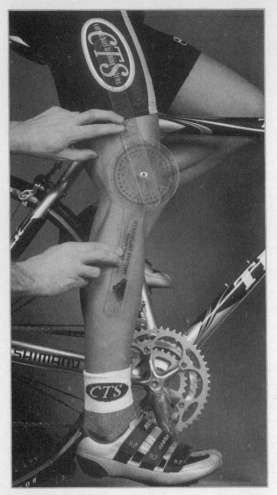

Measuring knee angle at Dead Bottom Center. *Photo © by Charlie Lengal III*

of the seat tube. It is suggested that you subtract three millimeters from your value if you are using clipless pedals.

Crank length has obvious implications for saddle height. Any change in crank length necessitates an equal change in saddle height. The length of a crank is usually stamped on the back of the non-drive-side crank. It is measured from the center of the bottom bracket spindle to the center of the pedal socket. There are many thoughts on crank length. Try to best balance the mathematical ideal with the practical. Practical issues include experience, riding demands, and musculoskeletal alignment. Crank length can be generally recommended as a function of frame size. Time-trial cranks are typically 2.5 to 5mm longer than your road-crank length.

4. Establish Saddle Fore/Aft

For your records: Measure your seat setback by lowering a plumb bob off the tip of the saddle and determining the horizontal distance

Crank-Length Recommendation

FRAME SIZE	CRANK LENGTH
≤ 54 cm	167.5–170 mm
55–57 cm	170–172.5 mm
57–61 cm	172.5–175 mm
≥ 62 cm	175 mm

from the string to the middle of the bottom bracket. You can mark your saddle rails where they meet the seatpost clamp.

Adjusting Fore/Aft Position:
Fore/aft placement of the saddle is a function of where the knee is over the foot when the crank is in the three-o'clock position. Pedal around a few times and stop in the three-o'clock position (crank forward and horizontal) with your foot as it would be if you were pedaling at about 90 rpm. Place the string of a plumb bob at the inferior (lower) tip of the kneecap. The plumb bob should intersect the pedal spindle and the

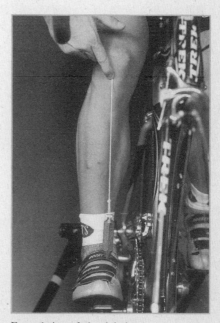

Frontal view of plumb bob.
Photo © by Charlie Lengal III

third metatarsal head. Saddle position should always be rechecked following other adjustments.

5. Establish Saddle Tilt

For your records: Place a bubble level on the top of the saddle and measure the tilt of the saddle using an angle finder.

Adjusting Saddle Tilt: Ideally, the top of your saddle should be level. Some people attempt to level the saddle by using a bubble level on the front and back of a saddle, but not all saddles are created equal. The level is a good place to start, but there are certain indications that the best position for a saddle may not always be level. Those indications include the necessity of fully extended arms, excessive pressure on hands, an arched back, and certainly excessive perineal pressure. Erik Moen recommends a simple sit-up test. With your bike level on a trainer, sit up and ride without the hands on the bars. If you feel like you are sliding forward, the nose of the saddle needs to come up. If you feel excessive pressure or numbness in the perineal area while you are riding with your hands on the brakehoods, the nose of the saddle should come down. If you are unable to locate a neutral tilt with these indicators, chances are the saddle will not work for your pelvic geometry.

Saddles come in all shapes and sizes, and replacing your saddle can inadvertently affect your seat height. Measure and record your saddle's length and its height from the rails to the top of the saddle.

6. Establish Handlebar Position

For your records: Since not all bars and brakehoods are created equal either, a measurement from the tip of the saddle to the tips of both of your brakehoods will give you an ultimate reach reference point. Variability in length of saddles, shape of handlebars, and placement of brakehoods make this measurement one of the only ways to ensure consistent reach.

Adjusting Handlebar Position: Handlebar position has large implications for comfort, aerodynamics, and handling. Your optimal reach to the handlebars is based on your hamstring/gluteal flexibility, trunk length, arm length, and core strength. Your goal is to achieve a trunk angle of 20 to 35 degrees (see photo, page 176). A common and effective method of finding a good stem length/height is to ride with your hands on the brakehoods and look down toward your front wheel. The bar and stem should occlude the front hub.

Your choice of stem length and stem rise significantly affects your trunk angle. Length of the stem is measured from the center of the steering column to the center of the handlebars. Rise describes the angle of the stem in relation to the steering column. A 90-degree angle between the steering column and the run of the stem is called a zero-rise stem. Rise stems are classified as positive-angle stems, and stems that appear flat or that dip down are classified as negative-angle stems.

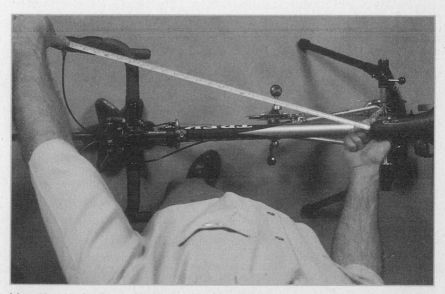

Measuring tip of saddle to tip of brakehood. *Photo © by Charlie Lengal III*

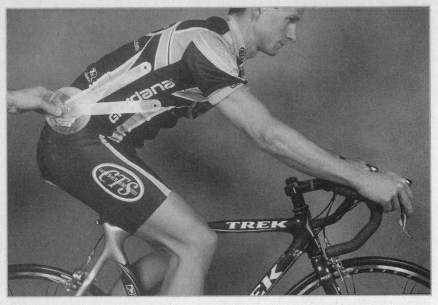

Measuring trunk angle. *Photo © by Charlie Lengal III*

7. Vertical Difference Between Saddle and Handlebars

For your records: This measurement should be taken using a level straight-edge projecting forward off the saddle, directly above the bars. Measure from the bottom of the straight-edge to the top of the handlebars.

Adjusting the Difference Between Saddle and Handlebars: Cyclists like to set up their bikes with high saddles and low handlebars, because that's what the pros' bikes look like. The problem is, most people don't have the flexibility and core strength to support that position. For some riders, this means raising the handlebars or shortening the stem. The table below provides guidelines for reasonable saddle-handlebar differentials, based on your height in centimeters.

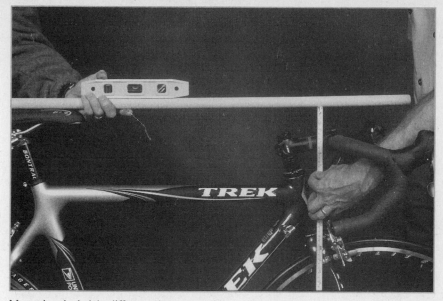

Measuring the height difference between saddle and bars. *Photo © by Charlie Lengal III*

Saddle-Handlebars Differential	
HEIGHT (CM)	**SADDLE-HANDLEBARS VERTICAL DIFFERENCE (CM)**
≤163 cm	0–2 cm
163–173 cm	3–6 cm
173–183 cm	4–8 cm
>183 cm	6–10 cm

8. Establish Brakehood Position on Handlebars

For your records: Handlebars are commonly measured by the distance between the drops, either middle-to-middle or outside-to-outside of the two drops. Make a second measurement at the brakehoods, as bars vary in style. This measurement is from middle-to-middle of the two brakehoods. With the bike perfectly level, measure from the lowest tips of the brake levers to the floor. They should be equal.

Adjusting Your Brakehood Position: The only rule here is to make sure you can get your hands to the brakes quickly and easily both from the brakehoods and from the drops.

Fitting the Time-Trial Competitor

The goal of a time trial position is to minimize your frontal surface area without compromising power production. You want to punch the smallest possible hole in the air and generate as much power as possible to push through it. Professional stage-race competitors and time trial specialists spend a great deal of time tweaking their time trial bikes and positions, seeking even the tiniest aerodynamic advantage. As an amateur cyclist, you need to ask yourself how many time trials you compete in each year, and how many of them are important goal events. Your answers should influence your approach to time trial equipment and positioning. If you rarely compete in time trials, you're better off using your road bike, as opposed to a time trial–specific bike, for events. However, if time trials factor heavily into your goals for the season, plan on spending more time and money on equipment, positioning, and practice.

Aero-positioning is valuable, as it can save you 10 to 40 seconds over a 40-kilometer time trial, but you need to practice to be able to compete effectively in an aero-position. Time trial positions tend to push your center of balance forward on the bike, and thus they change the way the bike handles. The long levers of the aerobars also influence handling. What seem like small steering changes at the end of your bar will make for larger

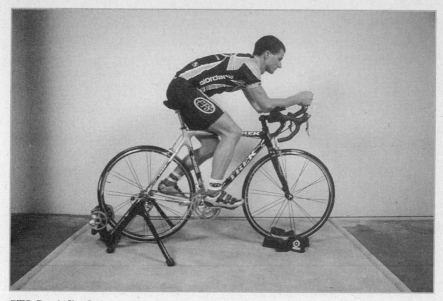

CTS Coach Jim Lehman demonstrates good time-trial positioning on a standard road bike. *Photo © by Charlie Lengal III*

changes at the front wheel. Be careful not to make your aero-position so extreme that it limits your power production or your ability to breathe.

The biggest difference between your road and time trial bikes is seat position. Rotating your position up and forward helps decrease frontal surface area and open your hip angle. As you reach for the aerobars, your hips roll forward on the saddle. If you don't move your saddle up and forward, you will close the hip angle, making it more difficult to pedal efficiently. Saddle tilt must also be changed, because a level saddle will not allow for a comfortable, flat-back aerodynamic position. You should tilt the nose of the saddle down slightly so you can roll your hips forward without causing excessive pressure in the perineal area. In the end, your knee angle at bottom dead center should very closely resemble that of your road position.

The simplest method of positioning aerobars is to measure your shoulder and elbow angles when you are in the aero-position. Your shoulder and elbow should both be at 90-degree angles. The extensions of the bars should be parallel to the ground and close together. Moving your arms closer together helps significantly with aerodynamics, but it

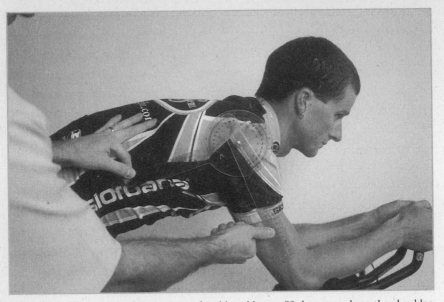

Place your aerobars so that you can comfortably achieve a 90-degree angle at the shoulder.
Photo © by Charlie Lengal III

also detrimentally affects breathing and your ability to steer. Experiment with the distance between your arms until you find a place where you can comfortably ride at high intensity.

Adapting a Road Bike for Time Trials

For those without a dedicated time trial bicycle, there are some important issues to consider when adapting a road bike for a time trial. Since you spend the vast majority of your time riding in your endurance position, make sure you can quickly and accurately reverse your time-trial modifications. Have a dedicated seatpost and saddle that you switch out for training or racing in your aero-position. It took you long enough to find an endurance road-saddle position; don't chance losing it.

If you rarely do time trials, consider a moderate aero-position that is not very different from your road position. This should resemble your on-the-drops position, because that is a position your body is relatively accustomed to. You will need to incorporate aerobars and mild position changes of the saddle/seatpost. Again, practice of the aero-position is important. Competing well in an aero-position takes practice. Plan on

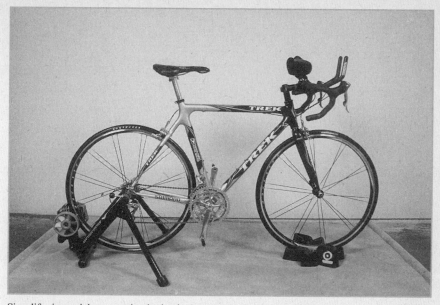

Simplify time-trial preparation by having separate seat/seatpost combinations. Note the difference in saddle position between the two pictures. *Photo © by Charlie Lengal III*

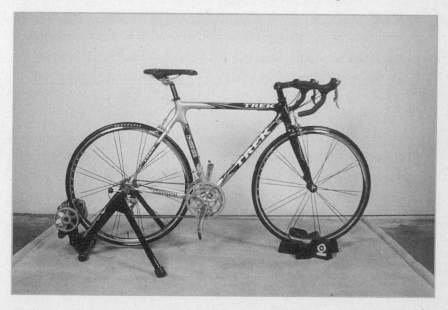

performing training workouts in your aero-position to ensure comfort, economy, and power production. Lance Armstrong trains on his time-trial bike at least once a week throughout the year, and almost always at high speed. It is important to be comfortable and confident with the way the bike handles at 50 kilometers per hour, so he spends time pacing behind a motorcycle on his time trial bike.

New Equipment

New equipment that may alter bike fit should be added only with some forethought. What will this new equipment do to your cycling position? Shoes and pedals are a good example. Different brands of shoes and cleats have different measurements between the pedal and the foot (the stack height). New handlebars may make your brakehoods mount farther away, thus necessitating a shorter stem. New equipment that may affect fit should be incorporated at a time when you can either adapt to a new position or have time to ensure good position. Never try new equipment under race conditions.

Keys to Adjusting Your Riding Position (on Any Bike)

1. You should never try a new position or equipment before or during a hard training ride or any race. Erik Moen comments, "I once worked with an athlete who had to sit out the middle of his competitive season due to a muscular-strain injury of the gluteus maximus muscle. He sustained the injury while competing in a time trial position that was new for him, and unfortunately it was a poor fit for his strength and flexibility."

2. Changes to position or equipment should be made during a time when your training volume and intensity are low. The Transition Period of training, fall and early winter, is a wonderful time to get used to a new position.

3. Change only one variable at a time, and allow a few days of riding before changing anything else. This way you can determine the effects of each individual alteration.

4. Changes in position must be made in small increments. Your muscles are very accustomed to their current ranges of motion. Drastic changes can lead to injury.

5. New positions oftentimes require changes in flexibility and/or strength. Will Frischkorn, one of the young professional cyclists I

work with, missed much of the 2001 racing season due to back trouble. Working with Andy Pruitt at the Boulder Center for Sports Medicine, Will made significant changes in his cycling position to better accommodate his back. Following the changes, it took several months of hard work for him to regain the power he had had prior to treatment. He went on to win the 2002 U23 National Road Racing Championship.

6. Adaptation to a new position may cause some discomfort. How much discomfort is too much? I have three criteria: it affects your ability to ride your bicycle; it lasts longer than 24 hours; sharp pains or numbness accompany each ride.

Positioning on the bicycle is important at any age; however, younger athletes (under 23 years old) generally tolerate position changes better than older athletes. The majority of the clients Erik Moen sees for bike-fit evaluations are middle-aged cyclists who are still trying to ride in the same positions they had 10 or 15 years earlier. Many of them have to accept the fact that age-related changes to the body may prevent them from riding comfortably in positions they used in their youth. It's better to raise your stem a little bit than to let pain force you off your bike for good.

THE RIGHT CLOTHES FOR ALL CONDITIONS

Cycling clothing has come a long way since the days when wool was the primary fabric for all seasons. Synthetic fabrics have made clothing more versatile, and what you wear can help you train effectively and race successfully. The human body can't tolerate core temperatures that are more than a few degrees above or below 98.6 degrees Fahrenheit (37 degrees C). Your body will use whatever energy it needs to maintain an acceptable core temperature, regardless of whether you would rather use that energy for training. Wearing the right clothing for the conditions reduces the stress on your body by helping to maintain optimal core temperature.

Layering your clothing allows for the right amount of insulation or ventilation for changing weather conditions. There are three main layers to consider when getting dressed to ride: a base layer, an insulating layer, and an outer shell. The base layer is the piece of clothing that is against your skin, and its main purpose is to move moisture away from your body. The evaporation of sweat is your personal cooling system, and fabrics that wick moisture away from your body assist in evaporative cooling when it is hot and prevent wetness from chilling you when it is cold. The insulating layer traps your body heat and keeps it close to your body, but it should be breathable enough to allow moisture to escape. During the summer, you probably won't use an insulating layer very often, but it is a staple of winter riding. An outer shell keeps wind and rain from reaching your insulating or base layers. The following table shows what fabrics to use in different applications.

Fabrics

	PROS	CONS
Base Layers (from best to worst)		
Chemically altered polyester (Capilene®, Thermax®)	Treatment makes the inside hydrophobic and the outside hydrophilic; pulls moisture to the outside away from skin	Holds odor
Polypropylene	Fibers let moisture travel away from skin while you retain body heat	Not as efficient at keeping moisture away from the skin
Wool	Tough, warm, and hardy	Retains moisture
Wool blend	Warm and comfortable	Good for lounging, but not a high-performance fabric
Polyester/cotton mix	Cotton's comfort and polyester's toughness	Minimal moisture-wicking ability
Cotton	Comfortable	Absorbs water and keeps it close to your skin

Fabrics *(continued)*

	PROS	CONS
Insulating Layers (from best to worst)		
Compact Synthetic (Thinsulate®, Thermoloft®)	Warm, very compressible, great performance when wet, dries quickly	Very few cons
Wool	Good insulator	Heavy and retains water
Pile (fleece)	Light, breathable, traps warm air while absorbing little water	Often too warm for prolonged exercise
Down	Great warmth, compressibility; lightweight	Bad for wet conditions, difficult for layering in cycling, expensive
Outer Shells (from best to worst)		
Windproof/waterproof (Gore-Tex®, Sympatex®)	Keeps water out, and is breathable to let sweat evaporate	Needs ventilation via slits, zippers, etc.
Windproof/water resistant	Keeps out some water, but is breathable to let sweat evaporate	Heavy or consistent rain will soak through
Nylon taffeta	Lightweight, windproof	Not waterproof
Polyester/cotton blend	Tight weave is wind-resistant	Neither windproof nor waterproof
Cotton	Tight-weave designs may shed wind	Absorbs water

George Hincapie learned the hard way that clothing can affect performance. In the 2002 Paris-Roubaix race, George and the U.S. Postal Service team were driving the pace when a cold rain began to fall. Instead of going back to the team car for more layers of clothing, George continued to ride. He forged ahead and ended up in the lead group with

50 kilometers to go. But riding for hours in soaking wet, cold clothing had forced his body to burn a lot of energy to keep his core temperature up, in addition to the energy he was using to pedal as hard as he could. That extra energy expenditure was very costly, and George bonked in the final 25 kilometers of the race and flipped into a ditch. Two things went wrong that day: George gambled that the time lost going back to the team car for clothing would be worse than the effect of the cold rain, and he didn't eat enough food to compensate for the increased energy he was burning trying to keep warm. In retrospect, the decision not to go back for clothing was beneficial to his position in the race, but it may have cost him a chance of winning Paris-Roubaix. As long as you remember to drink and eat enough, and don't let your core temperature fall too much, you can perform quite well in the rain and cold. Keep in mind that humans don't absorb a significant amount of moisture through the skin. No matter how wet you are on the outside, you still have to drink plenty of fluids to stay hydrated.

Hydration plays a large role in your ability to regulate your body temperature. The fluid volume for sweat comes primarily from the blood; therefore blood volume decreases as you sweat. If you don't adequately replace those fluids, blood volume falls to the point at which your body cannot both cool itself and support normal functions. As a result, you may stop sweating even though you are still working hard. This is known as heat exhaustion, and in severe cases it can be fatal. Heat exhaustion happens most often on hot and dry days, but the severe dehydration that contributes to heat exhaustion can occur in any weather conditions.

Your extremities are very sensitive to changes in body temperature. They lose body heat in cold weather before your torso does, and they are your body's radiators in the heat. In cold weather, your body constricts blood flow to extremities in order to preserve adequate core temperature. In hot weather, the blood vessels dilate to allow more blood to the extremities to dissipate excess heat. Your cycling gear should assist in these tasks to reduce the stress on your body.

The greatest amount of body heat dissipates from the head, so it is important to wear the right gear for the weather conditions. Research shows that new helmet designs actually help keep the head cooler than riding bare-headed or with a cycling cap. While this should not be the primary reason for wearing a helmet, it does invalidate the excuse that helmets are "too hot." In the winter, you should either cover some helmet vents, wear a cap under your helmet, or both. Your winter cap should also cover your ears to prevent frostbite.

CLOTHING TIPS:

1. It is better to slightly overdress than to underdress. If you are wearing layers, you can take one off if you get hot. If you're too cold, though, you can't put on more clothing unless you have it with you.
2. Save a layer of clothing to put on if you are going to be riding against a headwind on a cold day. While you ride with a tailwind, sweat tends to build up on the front of your body because there is less airflow to evaporate it. When you then turn into a headwind, the front of your body gets cold very quickly unless you have a wind-resistant layer to put on.
3. Gloves, arm and leg warmers, tights, and booties come in a wide variety of weights to provide the right amount of warmth for various conditions. Experiment to determine the clothing combinations that best fit the environment where you train.
4. Covering your knees is mandatory when the air temperature is less than 65 degrees Fahrenheit. The knee joint doesn't receive much blood flow in any weather, so it is one of the first places to get cold.

TAILORING YOUR TRAINING TO RACES

A proper training program makes you a complete cyclist, able to compete in any type of race. Even a track sprinter like Marty Nothstein trains as a cyclist first and a specialist second. Ask anyone who trains in the Trexlertown, Pennsylvania, area. Marty has been out doing long endurance rides, lactate-threshold intervals, and climbing workouts ever since he was a junior. He and I worked together before the 1996

Olympics because we understood that even in events as specialized as the Match Sprint and Keirin on the track, a stronger aerobic system makes a rider more powerful for all aspects of cycling.

Your training has to prepare you for of all types of racing, and then you can tailor your program to prepare specifically for a goal event. Stage racing demands different things of your body than criteriums do, but all success in racing is built on the foundation of a strong aerobic engine. It will be only during the Preparation and Specialization Periods that you begin to tailor your training to the specific demands of your chosen goal event.

Stage Racing

You need a huge aerobic foundation to handle consecutive days of racing in a stage race. Your training should prepare you to use your aerobic system for as much of the race as possible. This reduces the cumulative strain on your body so you can recover from day to day. With every effort over lactate threshold in a stage race, you are dipping into energy reserves that you will need tomorrow or the next day. Your training for a stage race improves your fuel utilization to allow you to spare as much glycogen as possible. This happens as a result of consecutive long training days, during which you are focusing on eating and drinking during and after the rides. Those habits have to become second nature so you maintain them when you are dealing with the stress of racing.

The 2002 Tour of Spain was Dave Zabriskie's first three-week stage race. In the months before the race, I included several blocks of consecutive long training days in his schedule. The goal was to improve his ability to recover enough overnight to handle the training the next day. The workouts were important, and so were his habits during and between training sessions. Dave had to be extremely vigilant regarding hydration and nutrition during rides, because dehydration and glycogen depletion make rapid recovery difficult. I slightly reduced the amount of VO_2 and sprint training in his program in order to increase the training load on his aerobic system.

The Tour of Spain was hard for Dave, and he contemplated dropping out. Johan Bruyneel wanted to see him complete it, as I did, because riders mature immensely by completing their first three-week

Tour. The first one is the hardest because it is a huge challenge with many unknowns. Dave called me after the first week of the race and said he didn't think he could make it to the finish in Madrid. He had been suffering for a week, and the prospect of two more unrelenting weeks was too formidable. I knew he had the physical ability to finish the race, and I had to get tough with him to convince him that he had what it took to finish. I told him that under no circumstances was he to pull off the course and stop. I didn't care if he was 30 minutes off the back, riding alone in a cold rain; he had to ride to the finish line each day. Dave is a talented rider who works hard, and his teammates and directors know that. They helped him out and looked after him, making sure his exhaustion didn't adversely affect his nutrition and recovery habits. He struggled through the second week of the race and adapted to the stress. Many times, a rider actually gets stronger in the third week of a Tour, and that experience bolsters his confidence in his ability to compete at that level. Dave adapted so well in the third week of the Tour of Spain that he finished 15th in the final time trial of his first three-week Tour.

To be a successful stage racer, you have to be efficient in every aspect of cycling. Race carefully, because any effort you don't absolutely have to exert is a waste of energy. Never give 100 percent unless you really need to; keep that energy in reserve for a moment of crisis. Going all-out for an intermediate sprint for 50 percent on the first day may come back to haunt you on the third day when you don't have the energy to catch the field after being dropped on a climb.

One-Day Racing

In some ways, a Spring Classic is harder than a three-week Tour. Since these races are winner-take-all, the intensity is extreme from start to finish. There are attacks, counterattacks, and extended periods of all-out racing throughout the race. You have to be able to handle repeated maximal efforts to stay with the lead group. Your training has to prepare you for repeated efforts with little or no recovery between them. George Hincapie excels in such races because his training includes hard interval sessions that mimic such demands. PowerIntervals, DescendingIntervals, and OverUnder Intervals are the best for developing the ability to attack again and again in hard races. The recovery between intervals is too short to allow for full recovery, and this trains your body to tolerate high levels of lactic acid while still producing maximal power.

The taper for a one-day race is longer than for a stage race. It is very important for a rider to be fresh for a one-day event. Often the taper starts two weeks before the race. Training volume decreases, but the intensity of individual workouts increases. The reduced volume allows you to recover fully between workouts, preventing the high intensity from leading to overall fatigue. I like to prescribe a very long ride about three days prior to a one-day race. This long ride depletes a rider's glycogen stores and applies a large stress on his or her energy systems. Following this workout, the rider benefits from a supercompensation effect. The body responds to the stress and depletion by stocking up on nutrients and priming the energy systems for another hard day. George Hincapie used this strategy in 2001 as he prepared for a week of racing that included the Tour of Flanders, Ghent-Wevelgem, and Paris-Roubaix. Three days before Flanders he rode for seven hours, including two hours of motorpacing (riding behind a car or motorcycle) at the end. The supercompensation effect helped him race to a 13th-place finish in Flanders. Three days after that, he benefited from the depletion caused by Flanders to win Ghent-Wevelgem. The taper for a stage race is shorter, because you don't want to erode any aerobic fitness in the process of resting up for the event. This is less of a concern for one-day racers, because they don't need to be able to race again on the following day.

Criterium Racing

Criteriums differ from one-day road races in that they are much shorter and involve more frequent maximal efforts. The training and taper for criterium racers are very similar to those for one-day road racers, but the week before the race is different. It is absolutely essential to be fresh and rested for a big criterium. I often skip the long depletion ride three days before race day. Criteriums are so short that the supercompensation effect that works so well for one-day racers loses its value. Races need to be more than three hours long to really benefit from supercompensation. On race day, your warmup is as important as your fitness for criteriums, because critical moves often happen in the first ten minutes of racing. You can't hide in the field for the first hour waiting until you feel good enough to make your move. As a rule of thumb, the shorter the event, the longer the warmup. If you are racing a 45- to 60-minute criterium, warm up for an hour. Many riders keep their warmups too short or too easy because they believe a longer or harder warmup burns too much of the energy they need for the race. Then riders who have arrived at the start line after long, hard warmups drop them in the first five laps. Your warmup has to have specific purposes. It has to be long and hard enough to activate all of your energy systems. You will be sprinting out of a corner at 35 mph within the first two minutes of racing, and your body can handle that only if you are primed to access your lactate threshold and VO_2 systems. If your warmup has only activated your aerobic system because you were cruising around the parking lot, you are going to get dropped. Over the years, I have developed a warmup routine that works well for most racers I work with. Try the following routine on a trainer or rollers before your next criterium and I believe you will find the first half of the race more manageable. You should use the power or heart-rate values you use during your workouts in the listed segments of the warmup.

Pre-Race Trainer Warmup
- 20 minutes EnduranceMiles (EM)
- 10 minutes Tempo (T), 75 to 85 rpm
- 2 minutes RecoveryRide (RR)
- 4 minutes SteadyState (SS), 90 to 95 rpm
- 2 minutes RecoveryRide (RR)
- 2 minutes PowerIntervals (PI), 105 rpm
- 2 minutes RecoveryRide (RR)
- 2 minutes PowerIntervals (PI), 105 rpm
- 2 minutes RecoveryRide (RR)

Total warmup time: 46 minutes

Get off the trainer as close to start time as possible. Try to get to the starting line warm and sweating. The warmup is used to get the body to produce lactic acid at an accelerated rate while beginning the buffering and clearing process. Your body will be primed for the intensity of the race start.

Time Trials

Time trials differ from all other types of racing in that the intensity is steady and unrelenting from start to finish. There is nowhere to hide, no draft to recover in, and no other racers to commiserate with. Your training has to prepare you for a sustained effort at and above your lactate threshold. This means not only long SteadyState workouts to increase your power output at lactate threshold, but also interval work to improve your lactate tolerance. OverUnder Intervals work well for this because you start the interval riding near threshold, increase your intensity to above threshold, and then return to riding near threshold. Your body adapts to continuing to ride hard even after you have accumulated lactic acid by riding above threshold. This adaptation is important, because it allows you to push above threshold during a time trial without having to drastically slow down to recover from the effort. People lose massive amounts of time due to short climbs in time trials. The climb forces them to ride above threshold for one to two minutes, and then they lose time because it takes five to six minutes for them to recover enough to produce the same power they were producing before the climb.

As with criteriums, time trials are so short that your warmup be-

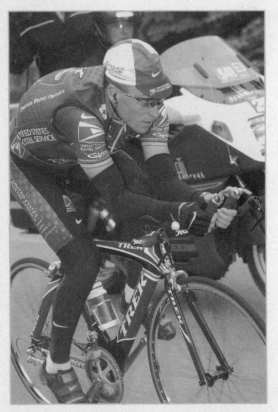

Lance Armstrong warming up for a time trial. He spends considerable time throughout the year training specifically for races against the clock. *Photo © by Graham Watson*

comes critical to your success. Typically, time trials in the U.S. are 40 kilometers or shorter and therefore take about an hour. The warmup routine provided earlier in the Criterium Racing section of this chapter also works well for time trials. If you ride a time-trial bike or modify your position on your road bike for time trials, make sure to train in that position prior to racing. On race day, warm up on that bike as well.

PREPARATION PERIOD TRAINING EXAMPLES

Your Preparation Period training builds upon the aerobic work you completed during the Foundation Period. Your endurance rides increase in pace as you progress from FoundationMiles to EnduranceMiles, and the intensity of your workouts increases from Tempo to SteadyStates. Consistency is very important during this period, because cumulative time at specific intensities is what leads to major gains. Try to ensure that you can complete an entire 40-minute Tempo interval without stopping for traffic lights or stop signs. Some athletes who live in urban areas complete the EnduranceMiles portion of the session outdoors, and then complete their interval work inside when they get home. The Preparation Period is also the time when you should be using hard group rides and training races to develop your early competitive fitness. By the end of the Preparation Period, you should be competitive in local and regional events, though not as strong as you will be at your peak.

Preparation Period Training Examples

	MONDAY	TUESDAY	WEDNESDAY	
Intermediate 5-Day				
Week 1	Rest Day	2hr EM w/4x5min MT	1hr EM	
Week 2	Rest Day	2hr EM w/5x5min MT	1.25hr EM	
Week 3	Rest Day	2hr EM w/40min T	1.5hr EM	
Week 4	Rest Day	1hr RR	1.5hr EM	
Advanced 5-Day				
Week 1	Rest Day	2hr EM w/6x5 min MT	1hr EM	
Week 2	Rest Day	2hr EM w/7x5 min MT	1.25hr EM	
Week 3	Rest Day	2hr EM w/65 min T	2hr EM w/55 min T	
Week 4	Rest Day	1.5hr RR	2hr EM	
Intermediate 6-Day				
Week 1	Rest Day	2hr EM w/4x5min MT	1hr EM	
Week 2	Rest Day	2hr EM w/5x5min MT	1.25hr EM	
Week 3	Rest Day	2hr EM w/40min T	1.5hr EM	
Week 4	Rest Day	1hr RR	1.5hr EM	
Advanced 6-Day				
Week 1	Rest Day	2hr EM w/6x5min MT	1hr EM	
Week 2	Rest Day	2hr EM w/7x5min MT	1.25hr EM	
Week 3	Rest Day	2hr EM w/65min T	2hr EM w/55min T	
Week 4	Rest Day	1.5hr RR	2hr EM	

	THURSDAY	FRIDAY	SATURDAY	SUNDAY
	2hr EM w/4x5min MT	Rest Day	2.5hr EM w/20min T	2hr EM
	2hr EM w/30min T	Rest Day	2.75hr EM w/45min RS	2.25hr EM w/25min T
	2hr EM w/30min T	Rest Day	3hr EM w/50min RS	2.5hr EM
	2hr EM w/3x12min SS	Rest Day	2.5hr EM	2hr EM w/3x10min SS
	2hr EM w/6x5min MT	Rest Day	2.5hr EM w/45min T	2hr EM w/6x5min MT
	2hr EM w/55min T	Rest Day	2.75hr EM w/60min RS	2.5hr EM w/45min T
	1.5hr EM	Rest Day	3hr EM w/70min RS	2.5hr EM
	2hr EM w/4x12min SS	Rest Day	2.75hr EM	2hr EM w/4x10min SS
	2hr EM w/4x5min MT	45min RR	2.5hr EM w/20min T	2hr EM
	2hr EM w/30min T	1hr RR	2.75hr EM w/45min RS	2.25hr EM w/25min T
	2hr EM w/30min T	1hr RR	3hr EM w/50 min RS	2.5hr EM
	2hr EM w/3x12min SS	1hr RR	2.5hr EM	2hr EM w/3x10min SS
	2hr EM w/45min T	1hr RR	2.5hr EM w/45min T	2hr EM w/6x5min MT
	2hr EM w/55min T	1.25hr RR	2.75hr EM w/60min RS	2.5hr EM w/45min T
	1.5hr EM	1.25hr RR	3hr EM w/70min RS	2.5hr EM
	2hr EM w/4x12min SS	1hr RR	2.75hr EM	2hr EM w/4x10min SS

7

A Champion's Nutrition Plan

PERFORMANCE NUTRITION VS. BASIC NUTRITION

Good nutrition is important for everybody; as humans we require a continual source of energy from food to perform all the complex functions of the body. The basic nutrients provide energy necessary to maintain our bodily functions both at rest and during exercise. Energy is needed for breathing, circulating blood, maintaining the body's core temperature, and the support of physical work. Nutrients—*carbohydrates, proteins, fat, water, vitamins, and minerals*—are essential parts of a complex process that takes place in the body to transfer the energy from the food we eat to our brain and body. These six classes of nutrients provide energy, regulate metabolism, and promote growth and development.

Athletes, however, can expend unusually intense efforts and large amounts of energy during training and competition, and this places great demands on their bodies. It is important to remember that it is common for athletes to have trouble balancing nutritional intake with the high demands of training. As an athlete, you place considerable demands on your body every day you train, recover, and compete. Too often, athletes spend all their time and effort training and working for top physical form, but ignore proper nutrition and rest. If you are not training with nutrition in mind, you are not getting the most out of your training.

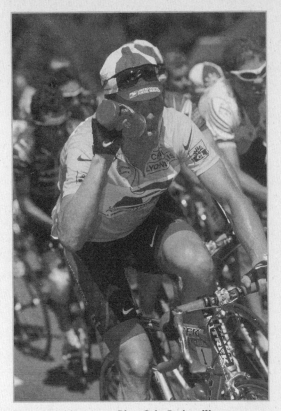

Lance drinking water. *Photo © by Graham Watson*

Just as the CTS training philosophy focuses on an athlete achieving the greatest benefit from the time spent training, the CTS nutrition philosophy focuses on an athlete achieving the greatest benefit from the foods he or she eats. Fueling the engine properly is critically important in working toward optimal performance.

Basic nutrition is the information you learned in grade school about the food groups and the necessity of eating a well-rounded diet. For the majority of the population, this is enough information to lead a healthy and somewhat active life. As a committed athlete, you are not in the majority of the population, and basic nutrition is not enough.

Athletes need to consider nutrition as a factor in performance. Performance nutrition, therefore, focuses on the effects of your diet on your training and competition capacities. Nationally recognized exercise guidelines say that 30 minutes of aerobic exercise per week promotes health. And while that is a true statement, it doesn't apply to you or your training goals. Likewise, nutritional guidelines written with the general population in mind don't apply to you either. You're an athlete with performance goals far beyond those of the general population, and as such, your diet needs to be based on performance.

QUALITY FUEL = QUALITY WORKOUTS

The aerobic system is the most critical element of performance; eating well is critical to ensure that your aerobic system performs at its best. A highly developed aerobic engine produces more energy from less fuel than any other system in the body. By selecting the proper foods as "fuel," an athlete can ensure he has the most fuel-efficient engine around. Think about putting low-grade diesel fuel into a high-performance car—the car may sputter and stall as you try to drive. However, with clean-burning fuel, the car would be able to operate at optimal efficiency, just as the performance of an athlete is optimized when the proper fuel is ingested. Not only are clean-burning fuels necessary for optimal performance and recovery, but good foods should be chosen to enhance overall health and well-being. As I talk in this chapter about the various fuels you can use for energy, I will also recommend quality sources and methods for obtaining the best fuel.

Optimal Fuel Mix
So what is the right fuel for the most efficient engine? Optimal physical performance requires a careful balance of essential nutrients. The energy, vitamins, and minerals from the foods we eat are essential to our ability to sustain physical activity. It is important to choose wholesome foods that are natural or lightly processed and have fewer additives. There are simple things you can do to shift to cleaner-burning fuel, such as selecting fresh apples instead of a sugar-loaded apple juice, and selecting breads and cereals made with whole grains rather than products made from refined flour. Look for whole grain—like 100 percent whole wheat—listed among the first few ingredients on nutrition labels. Natural foods tend to have a much higher nutritional value and fewer addi-

tives. Processing can add unwanted sugar and additives to food as well as strip away many of the essential nutrients.

Variety Is the Spice of Life

One other way to ensure that your engine receives the best fuel is to eat a wide variety of foods. No one food is a miracle food. Each food can offer its own special nutrients, and by eating a variety of foods through-out the day and from day to day, you can ensure that your body receives all the necessary nutrients. An athlete who eats a healthy diet, but who eats the same thing day after day, is actually robbing his or her body of the vast array of nutrients that are available. If cereal is a favorite break-fast option, simply eating different brands of cereal topped with a differ-ent fruit each morning can introduce a wider variety of nutrients to the diet. If a turkey sandwich is a favorite lunchtime meal, change the types of bread and condiments from day to day.

Fruits and vegetables are rich in carbohydrates, fiber, and many vita-mins, including health-protective phytochemicals. When thinking about fruits and vegetables in the diet, think *color*! When choosing a variety of fruits and veggies throughout the day, the color of the foods can give you a sneak peek as to the nutritional value. Usually the darker color a vegetable, the higher the nutritional value. For example, a deep green or deep orange means that there is more beta-carotene in a fruit or vegetable. Instead of munching on paler vegetables such as celery, mushrooms, or iceberg lettuce, choose darker-colored broccoli, squash, tomatoes, and carrots, which offer far more nutrients.

To optimize fuel choices, choose more of the best foods and less of the rest. If you can't think of one more way to eat spaghetti, try pasta in all its shapes and forms. Experiment with different types of rice and grains such as couscous and cracked wheat.

Carbohydrates

Carbohydrate is the body's gasoline—and your high-octane fuel. The reason for this classification is not only that carbohydrate is the most efficient form of energy during exercise, but also that it is the preferred fuel for most types of activity. While lots of hype is made about dietary protein and fat during exercise, carbohydrate is the primary fuel your body burns for energy. Carbohydrates are stored in the body as glycogen, and broken down to glucose, the fuel that allows you to train hard.

The body attempts to keep glucose levels constant, because it's the only fuel the brain uses. "Bonking" or "hitting the wall" is associated with a light-headed feeling for exactly this reason. When you bonk, there is still plenty of energy in the body to fuel muscles, but the brain is starving. The associated symptoms—nausea, headaches, poor coordination, confusion, and extreme fatigue—are more the result of your glucose-starved central nervous system than of energy-starved muscles. Bonking is a defense mechanism. Your brain is seeking to stop you from exercising so it can conserve fuel for its own survival. If glucose levels are low, the body protects the brain by manufacturing glucose from whatever's available—and in the absence of glucose it will cannibalize protein from your muscles. Therefore, it is important that athletes maintain an ample amount of carbohydrate in their daily nutrition; this is the best choice for fueling working muscles and promoting good health.

The quality and type of carbohydrate you ingest is critical to ideally fueling the aerobic engine. There are different kinds of carbohydrates available in many different types of foods. Major sources of carbohydrates include grains, breads, fruits, and vegetables. These clean-burning fuels include the energy needed for exercise along with a variety of *vitamins* and *minerals*—the spark plugs that your engine needs to run effectively.

Foods that are "nutrient-dense" supply a significant amount of nutrients per calorie. A high-performance diet emphasizes nutrient-dense carbohydrates necessary to maintain muscle glycogen—the primary fuel for cycling. Foods like whole-grain breads and cereals, rice, beans, pasta, vegetables, and fruits are considered to be nutrient-dense because not only are they high in carbohydrates but they supply other nutrients such as vitamins, minerals, protein, and fiber (see Table on page 202). By comparison, many refined and concentrated sweet foods, such as candy bars, doughnuts, and cookies, contain carbohydrates but are not considered nutrient-dense. They are high in fat and contain only insignificant amounts of vitamins and minerals. We refer to these types of foods as "empty calories." They provide the foodstuffs needed for a quick energy boost, but they can leave an athlete feeling tired and lethargic only 15 to 20 minutes after ingestion.

Nutrient-dense carbohydrates have another advantage over fats and sugary foods. Because they contribute significantly fewer calories for a given portion size than foods with a high fat or sugar content, nutrient-dense carbohydrates actually contribute to weight loss.

So how much carbohydrate is considered optimal for athletes? Sports nutritionists recommend that an athlete's diet consist of 55 to 65 percent carbohydrates, or 6 to 10 grams of carbohydrate per kilogram of body weight each day (kg/day). If you are training for an average of an hour a day, then your intake should be closer to six or seven grams of carbohydrate/kg/day. If you are training or competing for more than two hours a day, then carbohydrate intake needs to be closer to 8 to 10 grams of carbohydrate/kg/day.

Not only is carbohydrate necessary for energy *during* exercise, it is critical to ensure proper recovery *from* exercise. If you train hard on Tuesday and then don't take in enough carbohydrates after your workout, you will start Wednesday's training session with less than a full tank. This will not only affect your training session on Wednesday but also your recovery from that training session. As the days go by, you could actually be getting weaker instead of stronger! Adequate carbohydrate intake is critical to maximize training and recovery on a day-to-day basis.

A typical 150-pound athlete stores about 1,800 calories of carbohydrate—enough to support the first one to two hours of exercise at approximately a 70-percent-of-maximal effort. Training increases the ability of muscles to store carbohydrates (as glycogen) as well as improving the efficiency with which you burn fuel. As you become increasingly efficient in burning a combination of fat, protein, and carbohydrates during exercise, you prolong the time it takes to deplete your glycogen stores. In addition, taking in carbohydrates while exercising provides an additional source of energy that further extends the length of time you can exercise before running out of gas (more on eating before, during, and after exercise later).

High-Carbohydrate Foods

FOOD GROUP	CARBOHYDRATES (GRAMS)	CALORIES
Milk (higher percentage of simple carbohydrates; less nutrient dense)		
Chocolate milk (1 cup)	26	208
Low fat (2%) milk	12	121
Pudding (any flavor) (½ cup)	30	161
Skim milk (1 cup)	12	86
Yogurt (fruit-flavored, low-fat) (1 cup)	42	225
Yogurt (frozen, low-fat) (1 cup)	34	220
Beans (higher percentage of complex carbohydrates; more nutrient dense)		
Black-eyed peas (½ cup)	22	134
Garbanzo beans (chick peas) (1 cup)	45	269
Navy beans (1 cup)	48	259
Pinto beans (1 cup)	44	235
Refried beans (½ cup)	26	142
Fruits (higher percentage of simple carbohydrates; less nutrient dense)		
Apple (1 medium)	21	81
Apple juice (1 cup)	28	111
Applesauce (1 cup)	60	232
Banana (1)	27	105
Cantaloupe (1 cup)	14	57
Dates (dried) (10)	61	228
Grapes (1 cup)	28	114
Grape juice (1 cup)	23	96
Orange (1)	16	65

High-Carbohydrate Foods *(continued)*

FOOD GROUP	CARBOHYDRATES (GRAMS)	CALORIES
Fruits (higher percentage of simple carbohydrates; less nutrient dense)		
Orange juice (1 cup)	26	112
Pear (1)	25	98
Pineapple (1 cup)	19	77
Prunes (dried) (10)	53	201
Raisins (½ cup)	79	302
Raspberries (1 cup)	14	61
Strawberries (1 cup)	11	45
Watermelon (1 cup)	12	50
Vegetables (higher percentage of complex carbohydrates; more nutrient-dense)		
Carrot (1 medium)	8	31
Corn (½ cup)	21	89
Beans, lima (½ cup cooked)	20	108
Peas, green (½ cup)	12	63
Potato (1 large, baked, plain)	50	220
Pancake (4-inch diameter)	10	41
Pizza (cheese) (1 slice)	39	290
Popcorn, plain (1 cup, popped)	6	26
Pretzels (1 ounce)	21	106
Rice, white (1 cup)	50	223
Rice, brown (1 cup)	50	232
Saltines (5 crackers)	10	60
Tortilla, flour (1)	15	85

Protein

Proteins form the major structural components of all the cells of the body. They function as enzymes, membrane carriers, and hormones. The Recommended Daily Allowance (RDA) for both men and women is 0.8 grams of protein per kilogram of body weight per day. As an athlete, you need more protein than sedentary people do, but not nearly as much as we are sometimes led to believe.

One of the most common dietary mistakes I see athletes make is to supplement with too much protein. Some athletes have a protein drink after a ride or use protein shakes as snacks during the day. Although this is not harmful in itself, the intake of the extra protein usually comes at the expense of ingesting carbohydrate. One has to remember that carbohydrate is the main fuel source for working muscles during both riding and strength training. (Carbohydrate is the main fuel source for strength training because of its anaerobic nature.) In a normal state, when glycogen levels are high, the contribution of protein to energy is no more than 5 percent. Even in a starvation-like mode, when glycogen levels are depleted due to excessive endurance exercise or a poor diet, the contribution of protein as a fuel is 10 to 15 percent of the total energy.

Although carbohydrates are the main fuel source for cyclists, the slightly increased protein requirement for athletes is often due to the possible loss of protein muscle due to increased breakdown, usually after the exercise event itself, and because the body uses a small amount of protein as a fuel during exercise. A healthy recommendation is to keep protein intake between 1.2 and 1.7 g/kg body weight/day. Athletes generally meet the increased need by simply ingesting more calories to meet the increased energy-need demands. When athletes eat enough to meet their caloric requirements, they generally take in enough protein. Most athletes who eat a balanced diet with moderate portions of protein-rich foods will receive enough protein.

Sources of Protein Athletes can easily meet their protein requirements when their diets provide 12 to 15 percent of their total calories as protein. An ounce of meat, poultry, or cheese, or one egg, supplies about seven grams of protein with all the essential amino acids. Although animal products generally provide the highest-quality protein, slabs of steaks and juicy burgers have a very limited place in a healthy diet. By making choices that emphasize chicken or turkey without the skin, lean meat, fish, and nonfat or low-fat dairy products, you can meet your protein requirements and minimize the dietary fat.

1. *Lean Beef.* A lean roast-beef sandwich made with two thick slices of bread is an excellent choice not only for protein but also for iron, zinc, B vitamins, and other nutrients that are important for the sports diet. In terms of heart health, a lean roast-beef sandwich is preferable to a grilled-cheese sandwich or a hamburger because of these nutrients and the lower fat content. Top round, eye of round, round tip, and any other cut with "round" in the name are among the leanest cuts of beef.

2. *Chicken and Turkey.* Poultry generally has less saturated fat than red meat does, so it tends to be a more heart-healthy choice. White meat is leaner than dark meat and you should remove the skin, as it is very high in fat.

3. *Fish.* Canned or fresh, fish not only is a great source of protein, but may also protect your health. The best choices are the oilier varieties such as salmon, albacore tuna, swordfish, sardines, and bluefish.

4. *Plant Proteins.* You can eat a variety of plant proteins (beans, nuts, tofu, other legumes); however, you need to eat a generous portion of plant protein to equal the protein in animal foods. Peanut butter is a good source of plant protein, it has no cholesterol, and a few tablespoons on whole-grain bread, crackers, a bagel, or a banana offers protein, vitamins, and fiber in a satisfying snack or quick meal. Watch the amount of peanut butter in your diet, since it is high in fat and calories. A low-fat option may be found in almond butter or other nut butters. Go for the unprocessed, natural varieties, because they have more polyunsaturated oils. Tofu (soybean curd) is a vegetable protein that is easy to add to any diet. It has a mild flavor, so you can easily add it to salads, chili, spaghetti sauce, and other mixed dishes.

Protein's role in recovery is probably more important than its role in providing fuel for exercise. Not only does your body need protein to repair damaged tissue and build new cells, its presence immediately following exercise increases the uptake of carbohydrate into muscle cells. I'll cover that in more detail later in this chapter.

Fat as Fuel

Although fat usually gets a bad rap, it does serve many vital functions in the body, including providing an unlimited source of fuel. In addition, fat is an essential component of cell membranes, aids in the production of hormones, and also transports and stores fat-soluble vitamins in the body.

Unfortunately, fat also contributes to a number of potential health hazards. In fact, the amount and the type of fat eaten are associated with more major diseases than any other component of the diet. Carbohydrates are superior to fats for high-intensity events (both for training and on event day) and fats may, at their best, be equal to carbohydrates for lower-intensity, endurance events. Even the leanest athlete has plenty of stored fat available (approximately 38,000 calories' worth in a 154-pound male).

There are three major categories of fats: triglycerides (Tg), cholesterol, and phospholipids. Although phospholipids are important, Tg and cholesterol are of more concern in the diet. Triglycerides account for about 95 percent of fats consumed, while cholesterol constitutes only 5 percent.

Cholesterol and phospholipids are essential building blocks for cell growth, while triglycerides are used primarily as a source of energy. Triglycerides are what most people call "fat" in terms of food. They are the principal form in which fats are eaten and stored in the body. Excesses of saturated fats and cholesterol can contribute to obesity and heart disease, so being aware of the type of fat you are ingesting is as important as controlling the amount of fat in your diet.

A fatty acid is a component of a triglyceride. There are four types of fatty acids: two that are considered "good fats"—monounsaturated and polyunsaturated—and two very bad fats—saturated and hydrogenated. Although it seems like an oxymoron, there is such a thing as good fat. Of the many varieties of fat that can be found in foods, the more unsaturated a fat is, the healthier fuel choice it is for you. Fats derived from animal sources generally contain more saturated fat than those derived from plants. A healthier choice is monounsaturated or polyunsaturated fats.

Monounsaturated fatty acids

The more unsaturated a fat is, the healthier fuel choice it is for you. Monounsaturated fatty acids are liquid at room temperature and are derived from vegetable sources. Good sources include olive oil, canola oil, and avocados. There seems to be a health-protective effect from these types of "good fats." A decrease in heart disease has been shown when monounsaturated fatty acids are substituted for saturated fatty acids.

Polyunsaturated fatty acids

Like monounsaturated fats, polyunsaturated fats are liquid at room temperature and are derived from vegetable sources. The exceptions to this rule are coconut and palm oils, which are *very high* in saturated fats. Good sources of polyunsaturated fats include safflower oil, sunflower oil, and corn oil.

Saturated fatty acids

Saturated fatty acids are usually solid at room temperature and are most commonly found in animal products. They constitute the majority of the fat in many diets, including butter, lard, and the fat in whole milk, beef, pork, cream sauces, and ice cream. These are the least desirable form of fat from a health perspective. They can increase the level of low-density cholesterol (LDL, the bad one) and can facilitate the development of clogged arteries, strokes, and heart attacks.

Hydrogenated fats

Hydrogenation is a way of processing food that makes fat stay fresh longer, but the process changes the physical properties of fat, decreasing its health benefits. Monounsaturated and polyunsaturated fats, not saturated fats, are used in the hydrogenation process. In these types of fats, there are places at which oxygen can attack and damage the fatty acids. During hydrogenation, hydrogens are added to "fill up" these open bonds. Once an unsaturated fatty acid has been hydrogenated, it loses its health benefits and becomes a saturated fatty acid. When you read food labels, watch for ingredients stated as partially hydrogenated oils. These are saturated fats; stay away from them!

When making your food choices, one type of fat as compared to another will not necessarily impact your performance; however, the choices you make to support your athletic performance should also promote a healthy lifestyle. As an athlete, you should avoid highly processed foods that contain hydrogenated fats and are typically low in essential nutrients. By making choices that contain natural, monounsaturated fats, you not only increase the nutrient density of your diet, but also help to create a high-energy, heart-healthy environment.

Fat is used as a fuel during exercise of every intensity . . . not just light-to-moderate-intensity exercise. Studies have demonstrated that the intensity and duration of exercise, along with an athlete's training level and diet composition, all affect the composition of fuels used by muscles during exercise. The breakdown of fat to energy is a slow process that can only happen aerobically. Fat can supply about half of the energy for low- to moderate-intensity exercise; the majority of the rest of the energy comes from blood glucose and muscle glycogen. During

TYPE OF FAT	FOOD SOURCE	EFFECT ON HEART HEALTH
Monounsaturated	Olive oil, avocado, peanut butter, nuts and seeds	Desirable; will raise HDL and lower LDL
Polyunsaturated	Vegetable oils such as corn oil, safflower oil	Somewhat desirable; will lower HDL and LDL
Saturated	Palm kernel oil, coconut oil, animal products such as meat and butter	Poor
Hydrogenated	Processed foods such as crackers and snacks; margarine	Poor

higher-intensity exercise (greater than 70 percent of maximal VO_2), muscle glycogen will supply most of the energy, but fat still does contribute a small portion. During low-intensity exercise, fat is burned for fuel, but at a slow caloric burn rate. Even though there is a huge amount of fat energy in the body, carbohydrate is the primary fuel for exercise because the process of breaking glucose down into usable energy is quicker than the process for breaking down fat for energy.

Since carbohydrate stores are limited, the use of fat for energy production can delay exhaustion. One adaptation from endurance training is an increased ability to use fat as an energy source. Unfortunately, simply eating fat does not stimulate the muscle to burn fat. Instead, eating fatty foods tends only to elevate fat levels in the blood, and then the fats must be broken down to be used for energy.

Water

Making up about 60 percent of our total body weight, water is the most common nutrient of the body. Although it contains no calories, water is essential to life, especially during exercise. Drinking too little water or losing too much water through sweat can inhibit the body's ability to function at its full potential.

As the primary component of blood, water also transports glucose, fats, and oxygen to working muscles and carries away metabolic by-products such as carbon dioxide and lactic acid. Most important during exercise, water is essential to regulating body temperature by absorbing heat from working muscles and dissipating it via sweat. As your body's temperature rises, your sweat rate will increase to prevent overheating. During high-intensity exercise in a hot environment, water loss through sweating and respiratory evaporation can be as much as two to three liters per hour.

Don't wait for your thirst to kick in to keep on top of your water intake. By the time you feel thirsty, you are already entering the first stages of dehydration. The sensation of thirst is triggered by a high concentration of body fluids. When you sweat and your blood loses a lot of water, the sodium content of your blood rises. This triggers your thirst mechanism and tells you to drink. Unfortunately, by this time you are already dehydrated.

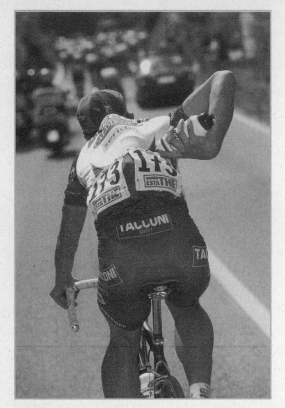

It's hard work supplying water to a team of thirsty cyclists. *Photo © by Graham Watson*

Being even slightly dehydrated can affect performance. Dehydration of only 2 percent (this means losing 2 percent of your total body weight in water) can impair your thermoregulatory ability. Less fluid in the body means less water in your blood; the measure of this is known as plasma volume. Once plasma volume decreases, heart rate increases in order to continue delivering enough oxygenated blood to tissues. With lower blood volume, the body retains more heat, so body temperature elevates. This will result in a decrease in the total work that your body can perform and will cause a dramatic decrease in time to exhaustion.

There is no other factor that impacts performance as greatly as hydration state. Most athletes could gain an immediate performance benefit by maintaining adequate hydration. The best way to accomplish this goal is to train with proper hydration and use a schedule. For example, set the timer on your watch to beep every 15 minutes to remind you to drink. Fluid needs during exercise are the same for men and women: four to eight ounces of fluid every 15 minutes.

A general rule of thumb is to drink enough water each day so that your urine is clear and odorless at least once a day, or you find yourself making trips to the bathroom every two to four hours. If your urine is dark, it means that it is concentrated with metabolic waste products and you need to drink more water. If you are always tired, have frequent headaches, and become sleepy often, this could also mean that you are chronically dehydrated.

Other beverages like coffee, tea, and soda add to your fluid intake, but do not contribute to your hydration needs. Since these fluids contain calories and other metabolic factors like caffeine, your body requires water to break them down. The caffeine in coffee, tea, and sodas can actually lead to more dehydration since they have a diuretic effect.

NUTRITION *BEFORE* TRAINING/ COMPETITION

It is well known in the cycling community that adequate carbohydrate stores are important for optimizing performance. It makes sense that eating carbohydrates before exercise can help top off your fuel tank and maintain blood-glucose levels during training and competition.

Since energy is derived from blood glucose, as well as from muscle and liver glycogen stores, it is important to maximize the fuel stores before exercise. Time for digestion is a major consideration when trying to figure out when and how much to eat before exercise. Numerous studies published over the last fifteen years have proven that eating 1 to 4.5 grams of carbohydrate per kilogram of body weight in the one to four hours before training or competition will maximize the available fuel during exercise. The carbohydrate and calorie content of the pre-exercise meal will need to be reduced the closer to the exercise session the meal is consumed. For example, an hour before training, a meal of 1 gm/kg would be appropriate, while a meal of 3 to 4 gm/kg would be better if you had four hours to digest the food before training or competition.

A major concern for many riders is what to do before an early-morning ride or race. When we wake up in the morning, we have essentially just undergone an eight-to-ten-hour fast. This overnight fast lowers the glycogen stores in the liver and greatly impairs the production of blood glucose. Since events lasting more than an hour rely heavily on blood glucose for fuel, performance will be adversely affected if you skip the morning meal. Waking up earlier to eat is one option, although the disruption of your sleep is probably more detrimental to your performance than de-pleted liver glycogen. Your other option is to eat a small meal containing both simple and complex carbohydrates. This combination will give you some readily available energy as well as some longer-lasting energy.

The pre-event food should be primarily carbohydrate with a touch of protein. Carbohydrate is the preferred fuel during exercise, and a bit of protein will aid with satiety. Be careful with your choice of high-protein foods, as many are also high in fat—bacon, cheese, and other dairy prod-ucts. Fatty foods should be avoided, as they delay stomach emptying and can contribute to feelings of sluggishness. Most important, never choose foods before competition that you have not tried in training! It's never smart to try anything new on the day of an important event. It may take some practice to determine exactly what your stomach can tolerate before a training session and how long it is going to take you to digest your pre-event meal.

Some good high-carbohydrate foods that work well for pre-exercise meals include fruit, cereal, bagels and bread, and low-fat or nonfat yogurt. Carbohydrates are digested quickly, increase blood glucose levels, and provide the best energy source for your soon-to-be-working muscles.

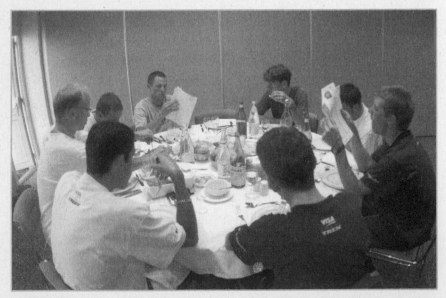

The U.S. Postal Service team sitting down to a meal during the Tour de France.
Photo © by Graham Watson

SAMPLE MENU FOR A 150- TO 160-POUND ATHLETE THREE HOURS
BEFORE COMPETITION:

> 2 English muffins
> 3 tablespoons jam
> 2 cups oatmeal
> 1 banana
> 12 ounces non-fat milk
> _____

TOTAL: 210 grams carbohydrate

SAMPLE MENU FOR ONE HOUR BEFORE COMPETITION (150- TO 160-POUND
ATHLETE):

8 ounces sports drink	8 ounces sports drink
1 energy bar	1 apple
½ banana	1 bagel

TOTALS: 70 grams carbohydrate   80 grams carbohydrate

NUTRITION *DURING* TRAINING/ COMPETITION

For training sessions or competitions that are going to last at least an hour, plan on consuming carbohydrates during exercise. Eating during an event is important for providing your muscles with fuel. There is enough stored glycogen in your body to go for 90 to 120 minutes at approximately 70 percent of maximal effort. After that time, when you do run out of glycogen, your intensity must drop as you use an increasing amount of fat for fuel. Research has shown that consuming carbohydrate during cycling can delay glycogen depletion and prolong exercise. Carbohydrate feedings have been shown to maintain blood-glucose levels when muscle-glycogen stores become depleted. What this means for you is that you can train longer, or sprint harder at the end of a race.

The secret for maximum performance in events lasting more than two hours is to eat every 20 to 30 minutes. A successful program requires striking a balance between eating enough to prevent hunger and avoiding the pitfall of the "if a little is good, a lot is better" philosophy. If one errs on the side of eating too much, there is the risk of stomach distention, bloating, and nausea. It is best to eat at the start of the event and continue with small amounts at frequent intervals. The key is to eat and/ or drink before becoming hungry or thirsty. Typically, the intensity of training or racing will prevent you from being able to replace enough fluids or carbohydrates during exercise to reverse the effects of glycogen depletion or dehydration.

To improve performance, a reasonable goal is to ingest 30 to 60 grams of carbohydrate per hour. This can be taken in as food, drink, or a combination of the two. Fifty-five to sixty grams of carbohydrate is equivalent to 16 ounces of a 6-to-8-percent-carbohydrate sports drink, or two PowerGels, or one PowerBar®. I remember when Brian Maxwell, founder of PowerBar®, and his wife were cooking the original bars in their kitchen and selling them at races. I've had a relationship with PowerBar® ever since, and we formalized that relationship in 2002.

Gels are specially formulated with a combination of simple and complex carbohydrates designed to provide quick energy during training sessions. They are intended to get sugar into your system as quickly as possible. PowerGels provide 100 calories (25 grams of carbohydrate) per packet, so you would need a gel packet every 30 to 45 minutes to provide the recommended 30 to 60 grams of carbohydrate per hour. Don't depend solely on gels for energy during long road races. Solid foods, such as sandwiches or PowerBars, are better in the early hours of a long event because they provide a longer energy burn and are less likely to cause intestinal distress.

NUTRITION AFTER TRAINING/ COMPETITION

Paying attention to what you eat after a training session or a race is equally important because it helps to replenish depleted muscle glycogen and shorten recovery time. Research has shown that muscle glycogen stores can decline on consecutive days of training if you don't pay attention to post-exercise carbohydrate and protein consumption. Consequently, adequate glycogen stores are essential not only for optimizing performance during competition, but also for maintaining the quality of training. By concentrating on eating high-carbohydrate foods after hard training or competition, you will be able to recover more quickly and be ready to train again sooner.

Athletes who wait more than one hour to consume carbohydrates re-store about 50 percent less muscle glycogen than those who consume carbohydrates during the one-hour period after exercise. Think of it as having more "doors" open into the muscle within the first 60 minutes af-ter exercise. Access to these doors to transport fuel back into your mus-cles decreases the longer you wait after a training session.

The optimal time to consume carbo-rich foods is within 30 to 60 minutes after exercise. Research shows that athletes increase their glycogen stores to greater levels than before exercise by eating foods high in carbohydrates within this time frame. By eating or drinking 1 to 1.5 grams of high-glycemic-index foods (recovery drink, white rice, honey, carrots) per kilogram of body weight immediately after exercise and every two hours for the next four to six hours, you will maximize glycogen stores. Since glycogen is the primary fuel for both on-the-bike and resistance-training sessions, replenishing your stores as quickly as possible is critical to maintaining quality training day to day. If you don't take advantage of the increased absorption rate, you will eventually re-store your depleted glycogen, but it may take up to 48 hours, and your training sessions in the following day will be affected.

After this initial four hours, muscle-glycogen stores are replenished at a rate of approximately 5 percent per hour. Although it may require up to 48 hours for complete muscle glycogen replacement after a two-hour ride, glycogen stores can be almost completely rebuilt in the first 24 hours. However, if you are training hard on back-to-back days or com-peting in a multi-day event, taking advantage of this window can be used to get a jump on the normal replenishment process and minimize the chance for chronic glycogen depletion.

Some riders take advantage of the post-workout window by using a recovery drink containing carbohydrate. Research has shown that there is NO difference in recovery between liquid supplements and a "real food" meal. However, if you are unable to eat a meal within that time frame, a liquid meal can be more convenient since you can ingest it anywhere. While it is beneficial to consume a recovery beverage within the first 15 to 30 minutes after exercise, it isn't enough to ensure that you will be ready to go again the next day. The 80 to 120 grams of carbohydrate consumed right after exercise gets converted to glycogen quickly, so it is also necessary to consume a high-carbohydrate meal within a few hours.

While protein is not as important as carbohydrate to fuel your workout, its role during recovery is very important. There is evidence that protein ingested within the first hour after exercise may help the absorption of carbohydrates. The most important part is not the protein itself, but its role in maximizing carbohydrate intake during this time. A four-to-one ratio of carbohydrates to protein is appropriate for muscle recovery. For every 100 grams of carbohydrate, add 25 grams of protein. One choice is cereal, a banana, and some skim milk for protein and carbohydrate.

Recovery Drinks

POST-WORKOUT SUPPLEMENT	AMOUNT	GENERAL EFFECTS
Carbohydrate	1.5g/kg body weight	Quickly restores glycogen Increases insulin concentration Increases growth-hormone concentrations Increases tissue absorption of testosterone
Protein	Only when added to carbohydrate	Increases protein synthesis Increases amino acids in bloodstream Slightly increases insulin concentration
Carbohydrate and Protein	4:1 ratio of carbohydrate to protein	Quickly restores glycogen Increases amino acids in bloodstream Increases protein synthesis Increases growth-hormone concentrations Increases tissue absorption of testosterone

Research has shown that protein, when combined with carbohydrate, almost doubles the insulin response and increases glycogen repletion after exercise. Insulin is a hormone that aids in the transport of glucose from the blood into muscle cells. It also stimulates an enzyme, glycogen synthetase, which governs the rate at which glucose is converted into glycogen. Increasing the insulin response increases the amount of glucose transported into muscle cells, and increases the rate at which it is converted into glycogen.

Protein can enhance muscle-glycogen replenishment, but that's just one part of the protein story. Protein provides amino acids, such as glutamine, necessary to rebuild muscle broken down as a consequence of exercise. For example, in Chapter 8, I'll talk about the role of the catabolic hormone cortisol in overtraining. Briefly, at the end of an intense training session, cortisol levels rise. Cortisol increases muscle-protein breakdown. Consuming a carbohydrate/protein drink that contains glutamine immediately after a workout or race can blunt this rise in cortisol, thereby reducing protein breakdown. Glutamine is also important for fueling the immune system. Low glutamine stores can suppress the immune system, making you more susceptible to colds and other infections during periods of hard training and competition.

Here's another bit of information that supports the use of a carbohydrate- and protein-containing post-workout drink: amino acids and dipeptides (found in whey protein) significantly increase the absorption of water from the intestines. Therefore, putting protein in your post-workout supplement may not only help replenish glycogen stores, it may also help with hydration!

CARBO LOADING: TRADITIONAL

As endurance athletes, cyclists rely on their stores of glycogen as a source of energy during competition. Carbohydrate loading is a legal method of boosting the amount of glycogen in the body prior to a competition. As we know, normal levels of muscle glycogen are more than enough to maintain exercise lasting less than 75 minutes; however, intensive training can deplete muscle-glycogen stores, increasing the need for carbohydrate intake to assure normal levels of blood glucose and sufficient muscle-glycogen reserves.

Research has found that carbohydrate-loading diets improve endurance athletes' performance. Traditional carbohydrate loading was accomplished in two stages: the depletion stage and the loading stage. During the first stage you would train to exhaustion in order to deplete muscle glycogen in your cycling muscles. For the next three days, you would consume a low-carbohydrate diet (60 to 120 grams of carbohydrate per day) while training moderately. During the loading stage, your diet would switch to a high-carbohydrate intake (400 to 600 grams of carbohydrate per day) for the next three days, while reducing training time. This would result in muscle glycogen "packing," increasing the muscle glycogen to a new, higher level.

A less stringent, modified carbohydrate-loading diet has been popular over the last decade. This modified regimen minimized some problems with the classic carbohydrate loading diet, including the disruption of training. The modified plan requires you to consume a 50-percent-carbohydrate diet for the first three days and then increase to a 70-percent-carbohydrate diet (or 4.5 grams per pound of body weight) for the last three days before competition. At the end of Day Three your body believes there is a problem with its glycogen stores and that it should store more glycogen than normal. In the last three days, when you consume carbohydrate and your training time decreases, your body replenishes glycogen stores and hopefully tops them up with a little bit extra.

Other research indicates that you may be able to build maximal glycogen stores in just a day. A speedier carbohydrate-loading regimen has been shown to help cyclists, runners, and other athletes preparing for events lasting longer than 90 minutes, while causing less disruption to their training. This method calls for a high-carbohydrate diet for 24 hours following a short bout of intense exercise. It also requires a massive amount of carbohydrate—ten grams per kilogram of body weight— and carbohydrate drinks are probably the best way to ingest that. A slice of bread averages 15 grams of carbohydrate. A 150-pound athlete would have to eat about 46 slices of bread to meet the target.

Whichever method of carbohydrate loading you choose, be sure to experiment with it in training. Some methods agree with certain athletes better than others do. And as always, you shouldn't try something new and untested for your goal event.

DIETARY SUPPLEMENTS (NON-FOOD)

Now that we've examined the effects of using "real food" to help support and enhance training, let's take a look at the use of dietary supplements that go beyond everyday food items. As an athlete, you place a high demand on your body. Manufacturers of certain supplements would like you to think that you can enhance your performance by using an array of vitamins, minerals, and other supplements. But how do you know what to believe? The $13-billion dietary-supplement industry boomed in the late 1990s, nearly doubling in size in five years' time. Being informed on what manufacturers are permitted to say, and knowing how to decipher the information on supplements' labels, can make you an informed consumer.

The Food and Drug Administration (FDA) traditionally considered dietary supplements to be composed only of essential nutrients, such as vitamins, minerals, and proteins. The FDA's definition of a dietary supplement includes:

> a product (other than tobacco) that is intended to supplement the diet that bears or contains one or more of the following dietary ingredients: a vitamin, a mineral, an herb or other botanical, an amino acid, a dietary substance for use by man *to supplement the diet* by increasing the total daily intake, or a concentrate, metabolite, constituent, extract, or combinations of these ingredients.

For decades, the FDA regulated dietary supplements as foods, in most circumstances, to ensure that they were safe and wholesome, and that their labeling was truthful and not misleading. An important facet of ensuring safety was the FDA's evaluation of the safety of all new ingredients, including those used in dietary supplements. However, with passage of the Dietary Supplements Health and Education Act of 1994 (DSHEA), Congress made changes that deregulated the industry and limited the FDA's powers. The actions that the FDA has taken against the most dangerous products are few and hesitant. Quality and safety standards are mostly voluntary and left to the discretion of the manufac-turer. As a result of these provisions, ingredients used in dietary supple-ments are no longer subject to the pre-market safety evaluations required of other new food ingredients or for new uses of old food ingredients.

"Dietary supplements" are now considered a separate regulatory category, and the DSHEA liberalized what information could be distrib-uted by their sellers. Consequently, manufacturers of drugs (many syn-thesized from plant compounds) must now generate research (clinical trials) to prove that a drug is not only safe but also effective. Unfortu-nately, the makers of dietary supplements still enjoy exemption from such legislation, and thus have no such requirement. In other words, makers of supplements don't have to prove that their products are either safe or effective. Instead, this new law shifted the burden of proof of supplement safety from the manufacturer to the FDA. Now this agency must prove the product unsafe before removing it from the market. Fur-thermore, when it comes to the efficacy of the supplement, the manu-facturers can say what they wish, so long as they do not claim that their supplement can prevent, treat, or cure a disease.

In January 2000, the FDA published a revised final rule on health claims for dietary supplements. DSHEA permits claims that products af-fect the structure or function of the body, provided the manufacturer has substantiating documents on file. Without prior FDA review, products may not bear a claim that they can prevent, treat, cure, mitigate, or diag-nose disease. The final rule still prohibits express disease claims (such as "prevents osteoporosis") and implied disease claims ("prevents bone fragility in postmenopausal women"). The new rule permits health-maintenance claims ("maintains a healthy circulatory system"); other non-disease claims ("for muscle enhancement," "helps you relax"); and claims for common, minor symptoms associated with pregnancy, meno-pause, or other life stages (e.g., "for common symptoms of PMS," "for hot flashes"). The nutritional-support statements must be followed by the phrase "This statement has not been evaluated by the FDA. This product is not intended to diagnose, treat, or prevent disease."

All of this leads to one major conclusion: let the buyer beware. If a company's claims sound too good to be true, they most likely are. Most athletes want to believe that there is a magic pill or potion that can help give them that extra edge, and manufacturers use that to manipulate consumers. When trying to evaluate whether a supplement can be beneficial, ask yourself the following questions to help evaluate the claims:

> *Is the person or company making the claims reputable? Is the only reason they are telling me about their product to sell me their product?* Be aware of statements that promise to dramatically enhance performance or guarantee fast results. Is their "ad" based on personal testimonials rather than scientific evidence?

> *What evidence is supplied for the claims that are made?* All claims should be supported with studies published in peer-reviewed, scientific journals. If you are uncertain, look up the study to be sure it is recent, and what the study actually investigated. Some "facts" get stretched or oversimplified to help support claims by manufacturers.

> *Do the recommendations conflict with most recommendations from sports science and nutrition professionals?* While there are breakthroughs and new ideas in the sciences of nutrition and supplementation, be cautious about anything that significantly opposes the facts of basic sports science and sports nutrition. If a manufacturer is recommending use of a supplement that eliminates certain foods or limits intake of others, you should be cautious.

So the big question is "Do athletes really need dietary supplements?" My answer is that a lot of people can benefit from moderate supplementation, but that not everyone needs it. A supplement should be taken when you are not ingesting enough of a nutrient through diet alone, but it is important to have your diet analyzed by a professional to determine if you have deficiencies. Besides correcting deficiencies, Dr. Ed Burke used to recommend taking a multivitamin as a "nutritional insurance policy." Your body will use what it needs and excrete the rest. Taking a multivitamin daily is a good insurance policy, but drastically increasing the dose rarely provides additional benefit and may be harmful. Iron and the fat-soluble vitamins (A, D, E, and K) are toxic at high doses.

Just as an effective training program that includes the right workouts, at the appropriate intensity, and in the right order leads to positive results, a high-performance diet starts with a meal plan. Included below are three examples of three-day meal plans, encompassing 2,000-, 2,500-, and 3,000-calorie-per-day diets. Please understand, these are only examples of the types of foods and general quantities that can make up these diets.

In order to determine which meal plan is appropriate for you, you first need to know how much energy you expend each day. It takes a certain amount of energy to maintain the normal functions of the human body, which is often referred to as your resting metabolic rate (RMR). Activities of daily life, like brushing your teeth, working at your job, cooking, and cleaning occupy their own category in the calculation of your total daily energy expenditure. The first two factors in energy expenditure remain relatively constant from day to day, although they gradually increase or decrease with changes in activity level, training status, lean body mass, and age. The big variable in your energy calculations is your activity level—the amount of energy you burn during exercise. Depending on your training, you could burn 4,000 calories or only a few hundred for a given day. Your total daily energy expenditure is a combination of your resting RMR, your daily activities, and your exercise level.

Resting metabolic rate is affected by your physical size, age, and training status. It generally increases as people get bigger, and decreases as they get older. Training leads to an increase in lean body mass, which in turn increases your RMR. A small, highly trained athlete may have an RMR equal to or higher than that of a less-fit individual much larger than himself. When you also factor in variations in people's daily activity levels (for example, sitting in a cubicle vs. moving boxes in a warehouse), and the constantly changing demands of exercise, it becomes difficult to use general formulas to determine your total daily energy expenditures.

My first recommendation is to seek the assistance of a sports nutritionist or registered dietitian (RD). These professionals can accurately determine the number of calories you need in order to stay healthy and perform at your best. Another way you can get some answers on your own is to record everything you eat for three days and use one of many free online dietary-recall calculators. These calculators will tell you your caloric intake, and if you are neither gaining nor losing weight, you can consider the caloric intake numbers from the online calculator a good estimate of which meal plan is right for you. Online calculators, however, offer information that is far more generalized than what you will receive from a sports nutritionist or RD, especially regarding the ratios of carbohydrate to protein and fat in your diet.

2,000 Calories-Per-Day Meal Plan

Average calories per day: 2,006
Average carbohydrate/protein/fat ratio: 63/20/17

DAY 1

Breakfast: Two bran muffins, one tablespoon of fruit preserves, and 1.5 cups of orange juice

Midmorning Snack: One bagel (approx. four-inch diameter) with one tablespoon peanut butter

Lunch: One turkey sandwich, a piece of fresh fruit, and a cup of cranberry juice

Afternoon Snack: Mixed nuts

Dinner: Tuna-stuffed pita with lettuce and tomato, one bowl of tomato soup, and a piece of fresh fruit

Basic Nutritional Summary:
Carbohydrate/protein/fat ratio: 66/17/17

CALORIES	PROTEIN	CARBS	FAT	SAT. FAT	SODIUM
1931	86 g	329 g	39 g	5 g	2272 mg

DAY 2

Breakfast: One honey-wheat bagel with two tablespoons of margarine and 12 ounces of fruit smoothie

Midmorning Snack: One medium-sized baked potato with half a cup of tomato salsa

Lunch: One barbecue-chicken sandwich with lettuce and low-fat blue cheese dressing, and a piece of fresh fruit

Afternoon Snack: One double-chocolate Powerbar Pria bar

Dinner: One bean-and-roasted-red-pepper burrito and half a cup of roasted-bell-pepper salad

Basic Nutritional Summary:
Carbohydrate/protein/fat ratio: 58/21/21

CALORIES	PROTEIN	CARBS	FAT	SAT. FAT	SODIUM
2,050	108 g	303 g	49 g	15 g	3,040 mg

DAY 3

Breakfast: Two egg-white crêpes and one cup of orange juice

Midmorning Snack: One ounce of low-fat cheese with crackers and a piece of fresh fruit

Lunch: One turkey sandwich on multi-grain bread, 1.5 cups of salad with low-fat dressing, and a piece of fresh fruit

Afternoon Snack: One 4.4-ounce container of yogurt (any flavor) mixed with granola and fruit

Dinner: Chicken chef salad (3 cups) with low-fat dressing, two dinner rolls, and strawberry shortcake (one cup of strawberries)

Basic Nutritional Summary:
Carbohydrate/protein/fat ratio: 60/27/13

CALORIES	PROTEIN	CARBS	FAT	SAT. FAT	SODIUM
2,037	142 g	322 g	31 g	2 g	2,900 mg

2,500 Calorie-Per-Day Meal Plan

Average calories per day: 2,536
Average carbohydrate/protein/fat ratio: 60/24/16

DAY 1

Breakfast: Two egg-white crêpes and one cup of orange juice
Midmorning Snack: One ounce of low-fat cheese, crackers, and piece
of fresh fruit
Lunch: One bean-and-roasted-pepper burrito, 1.5 cups of salad with
low-fat dressing, and one 4.4-ounce container of yogurt (any
flavor)
Afternoon Snack: One 4.4-ounce container of yogurt (any flavor)
mixed with granola and fruit, and one chocolate bar
Dinner: Chicken chef salad (3 cups) with low-fat dressing, two dinner
rolls, and strawberry shortcake (one cup of strawberries)

Basic Nutritional Summary:
Carbohydrate/protein/fat ratio: 61/23/16

CALORIES	PROTEIN	CARBS	FAT	SAT. FAT	SODIUM
2,605	157 g	416 g	47 g	10 g	4,131 mg

DAY 2

Breakfast: 1.5 cups of multi-grain cereal with raisins and non-fat
milk, and one cup of orange juice
Midmorning Snack: One PowerBar®
Lunch: One Greek pita sandwich with vegetables, six ounces of hum-
mus, and one ounce of feta cheese. One single-serving package
of non-fat pretzels and one piece of fresh fruit
Afternoon Snack: One 16-ounce fresh-fruit smoothie

Dinner: One medium-sized potato prepared with green and red bell peppers and six ounces of roasted chicken, a bowl of vegetable and lentil soup, and half a cup of yogurt (any flavor)

Basic Nutritional Summary:
Carbohydrate/protein/fat ratio: 63/22/14

CALORIES	PROTEIN	CARBS	FAT	SAT. FAT	SODIUM
2,463	144 g	412 g	41 g	10 g	3,093 mg

DAY 3

Breakfast: One bagel (approximately four-inch diameter), one ounce of low-fat cream cheese, and half a grapefruit

Midmorning Snack: One 4.4-ounce container of yogurt (any flavor) mixed with granola and fruit

Lunch: One serving of vegetable two-topping pizza (2 slices), one cup of spinach salad with low-fat dressing, and a piece of fresh fruit

Afternoon Snack: One single-serving package of baked tortilla chips and one chocolate PowerBar®

Dinner: Six ounces of beef-and-vegetable stir-fry over one cup of rice, two-thirds of a cup of yogurt

Basic Nutritional Summary:
Carbohydrate/protein/fat ratio: 61/26/12

CALORIES	PROTEIN	CARBS	FAT	SAT. FAT	SODIUM
2,450	169 g	393 g	35 g	89 g	3,654 mg

3,000 Calorie-Per-Day Meal Plan

Average calories per day: 2,961
Average carbohydrate/protein/fat ratio: 62/22/16

DAY 1

Breakfast: Two bran muffins with one tablespoon of fruit preserves, eight ounces of yogurt (any flavor), and 1.5 cups of orange juice

Midmorning Snack: One bagel (approximately four-inch diameter) with two tablespoons of peanut butter, and one cup of fruit juice

Lunch: One turkey sandwich and a bowl of vegetable, lentil, and barley soup, one piece of fresh fruit and one cup of fruit juice

Afternoon Snack: One PowerBar®, an ounce of mixed nuts, and one cup of fruit juice

Dinner: Tuna-stuffed pita with lettuce and tomato, one bowl of tomato soup with crackers, and a piece of fresh fruit

Basic Nutritional Summary:
Carbohydrate/protein/fat ratio: 66/18/16

CALORIES	PROTEIN	CARBS	FAT	SAT. FAT	SODIUM
2,969	136 g	511 g	55 g	8 g	3,194 mg

DAY 2

Breakfast: One bagel with two tablespoons of margarine and one 16-ounce fruit smoothie

Midmorning Snack: One medium-sized baked potato with half a cup of tomato salsa

Lunch: Barbecue-chicken sandwich with lettuce and low-fat blue cheese dressing, one piece of fresh fruit, and one PowerBar®

Afternoon Snack: One 4.4-ounce container of yogurt (any flavor) mixed with granola and fruit

Dinner: One bean-and-roasted-red-pepper burrito, half a cup of roasted-bell-pepper salad, and half a cup of frozen yogurt

Basic Nutritional Summary:
Carbohydrate/protein/fat ratio: 60/19/21

CALORIES	PROTEIN	CARBS	FAT	SAT. FAT	SODIUM
2,954	142 g	456 g	69 g	20 g	3,911 mg

DAY 3

Breakfast: Two egg-white crêpes and one cup of orange juice
Midmorning Snack: One ounce of low-fat cheese with crackers and a piece of fresh fruit
Lunch: One chicken-salad sandwich on multi-grain bread, 1.5 cups of salad with low-fat dressing, one piece of fresh fruit, and one single-serving package of non-fat pretzels
Afternoon Snack: One 4.4-ounce container of yogurt (any flavor) mixed with granola and fruit, and one chocolate PowerBar®
Dinner: Six ounces of baked chicken breast, two dinner rolls, 1.5 cups of chicken chef salad with low-fat dressing, and strawberry shortcake (one cup of strawberries)

Basic Nutritional Summary:
Carbohydrate/protein/fat ratio: 60/28/12

CALORIES	PROTEIN	CARBS	FAT	SAT. FAT	SODIUM
2,960	216 g	455 g	40 g	4 g	4,721 mg

8

Putting It All Together

T HE FOCUS AND SCOPE of your training really begins to narrow as
you move from the Preparation Period to the Specialization Period.
The biggest portion of the work has already been done. You have a
huge aerobic engine and more power at lactate threshold than ever before. You are maintaining a healthy weight and diet, and you have a positive outlook on training because of the short- and mid-term goals you
have accomplished. Your fitness and racing prowess are at the point at
which you are competitive in events and comfortable in racing situations. Things are going well, and you could maintain this level of performance for a long period of time, but to achieve your dream goal you
need to bind all of these different aspects of performance tightly together to support the effort required to achieve something greater than
you have ever achieved in athletics.

The difference between being fit to race and being fit to win can
come down to how well the various parts of your training enhance one
another. Eating a good, well-balanced diet is a good thing, but make sure

that the diet is actually enhancing your training by supplying the specific nutrients, in the optimal quantities, to replenish what your training is consuming. A good diet and a good training program together can lead to results greater than the sum of these parts. While I believe the parts of training ought to be balanced throughout the entire year, it is increasingly important during the Specialization Period because there is no time left to make drastic changes on the route to your goal.

Your training progress is maneuverable, but it's a vehicle that handles more like an oil tanker than a sports car. You can correct for periods when training interruptions, poor diet, or decreased motivation lead your progress off-course, but only if there is enough room to change direction and enough time to speed up or slow down. The Specialization Period is like pulling into harbor after crossing the ocean. You may have swerved your way through the open ocean, but now that you are close to port, every detail counts. Even the best captains defer to an experienced harbor pilot to guide them safely to where they need to go. Optimal performance is in the details, and during the Specialization Period both you and your coach have to monitor and adjust training daily to ensure that you arrive where you want to be, when you want to be there.

The Specialization Period usually begins about eight weeks prior to your goal event, and I don't recommend that it be any longer than 12 weeks. It is possible to have two Specialization Periods during the season, with some Preparation Period training between them to fortify the aerobic system. I'll discuss that process later in the book. For now, you need to understand that this period is a delicate balance between very hard workouts and a great deal of rest. During these workouts, the training load on your energy systems is huge, and the frequency and overall volume of training must decrease to give you enough recovery time between sessions. The workouts are shorter, and the time between them is greater to allow for maximum effort and full recovery.

Many athletes struggle to maintain a good balance between effort and recovery during the Specialization Period because they feel so strong on the bike. It is important to resist the urge to test your strength frequently, because doing so increases your training load and the recovery time needed between rides. Instead of being in peak condition for your goal event, you'll burn through the fitness you have and your performance will begin to decline before the big day. You don't want your best performance to be during training races and group rides three weeks prior to your goal event. Think of your strength as a precious and expendable commodity, and be judicious in the way you use it. You can use your strength and power to beget even more power, but only if you stick with your training program through the entire Specialization Period.

FIELD TEST TO CONFIRM PROGRESS

I believe in using a field test to confirm that an athlete has the requisite power to begin the Specialization Period. What I am looking for is the ability to maintain equal power outputs during the two time trials that make up the CTS Field Test, and in the absence of power information I look for the ability to maintain equal elapsed times for the two efforts. I judge an athlete to have good repeatability when he or she exhibits less than a 5-percent drop in power or speed from the first to the second field-test effort. Repeating equal times or power outputs indicates that an athlete has a highly developed aerobic engine, capable of supplying the majority of the energy for the effort. When the aerobic engine is less developed, the anaerobic system contributes more energy and leads to higher levels of lactic acid in the blood. When this is the case, the second time trial is slower or at a lower power output because the lactic acid hinders performance. The second performance marker I look for is a higher power output or faster elapsed time than during previous field tests. This indicates that the LT work from the Preparation Period has been effective in increasing the athlete's sustainable workload.

Your field test must adapt with your fitness level. Depending on your fitness and experience level, you may need to increase the length of the field-test efforts in order to judge your physical development accurately. The standard CTS Field Test consists of two three-mile (five-kilometer) efforts, but experienced and national-class athletes often need to adapt the field test in consideration of their fitness. For instance, I prescribe two ten-kilometer efforts for 2002 U23 National Champion Will Frischkorn because for him the five-kilometer test is too short. He has the power to complete two five-kilometer tests with absolutely equal times and power outputs at any time of year. But when I increase the length of the efforts to ten kilometers, the first effort takes enough out of him that the second effort pushes him to his limit. When Will is ready to start his Specialization Period, he can maintain very high and equal power outputs for two longer efforts, but during the earlier portions of the year, his power decreases during the second effort. When you can complete your second five-kilometer field-test effort with energy to spare, and if you feel like you could complete a third effort if you needed to, it is time to increase the length of your field-test.

Climbing field tests and flat-ground field tests are equally effective, although the results are difficult to compare. The heart rate, power, and elapsed-time information will be significantly different between the two environments. Your field tests provide a baseline to compare against current information, so consistency is important. You can utilize both types of tests during the year, but climbing field tests should be judged against previous climbing field tests, and flat-ground tests against previous flat-ground tests.

CONFIDENCE-BUILDING ACTIVITIES

A good field test can confirm that your training is on track, but it takes more than great conditioning to win bike races. It is important to confirm your race fitness with a real-world test in competition. By the end of the Preparation Period, you should be able to race competitively on a local and regional level. You may not be winning every race you enter, but you're not struggling to finish, either. In the beginning of the year, you established action goals (short term), confidence-building goals (midterm), and dream goals (long-term). One of the confidence-building goals you should have established was a race scheduled to coincide with the beginning of your Specialization Period. Choose a challenging race that has some similarities to your goal event; don't try to boost your confidence artificially by winning a short, easy race that no one else shows up for. This shouldn't be just another weekend race that you train through; this is a goal event that should be specifically prepared for, including a short taper. You don't have to win the race for it to effectively serve as a confidence-building activity. Just look at Lance Armstrong. He used the Amstel Gold Race as a confidence-builder from 1999–2003 and didn't win the race in any of those years. The events still served their purposes because Lance was a factor in the races, rode aggressively, and made all the right moves (with the exception of the finishes). His performances indicated to me that his conditioning and his racing skills were exactly where they needed to be on the route to ultimate readiness for the Tour de France in July.

The Specialization Period can be up to three months long, and your confidence-building race should be at least eight weeks prior to your goal event. Part of the reason Lance and I choose the Amstel Gold Race as a confidence-building event is that it is 10 to 12 weeks prior to the Tour de France and it coincides with the beginning of his Specialization Period. If I see indications that Lance's fitness isn't where it needs to be in April, I still have enough time to change his training plan and ensure he is 100% ready for the Tour de France in July. The Tour of Switzerland, which is usually three weeks prior to the Tour de France, is a bad time to find out that your athlete is behind schedule. At that point there isn't enough time to catch up before the Tour de France starts.

USING TRAINING DIARIES TO TRACK PROGRESS

The philosopher George Santayana once stated, "Those who cannot remember the past are condemned to repeat it." A good training diary details the progress and setbacks you have experienced over extended periods of time so you can repeat the good things you did and change the things that didn't work. Your goal with a training diary is to derive trends from the information you record, so data has to be consistent from day to day. I recommend dividing your diary into three sections: Training Data, Baseline Data, and Personal Data.

Training Data: What Did You Do Today?
Your training data consists of the details that describe your daily workouts. When you review this information later, you should be able to

determine accumulated hours of training, the amount of time spent at different intensities, and the number of training sessions targeted at specific systems and skills. Over time, you can identify trends in power output, training load, and other performance markers. The information to record in your Training Data section each day is:

Training Hours (entire workout)
Distance Ridden (optional)
Average Heart Rate (entire workout)
Average Power Output (entire workout)
Average Cadence (entire workout)
Specific Task(s) within the workout (i.e., Tempo, SteadyState Intervals, FastPedal, PowerIntervals)
Number of Interval Sets
Number of Intervals
Time of Each Interval
Recovery Time Between Each Interval
Recovery Time Between Interval Sets
Average Power of Each Interval
Average Heart Rate of Each Interval
Average Cadence of Each Interval
Subjective Comments About the Workout (Did the workout feel abnormally hard? Did you feel like you were pedaling through peanut butter, or were you floating on the pedals? Did you accomplish the goal of the workout? Did you have a good training day?)

Baseline Data: How Are You Handling Your Workload?

Baseline Data is information that helps you and your coach evaluate how well your body is dealing with your training load and recovery habits. There is a strong correlation between the work you do on the bike and basic bodily functions off the bike. Baseline data stays relatively constant throughout the year, and deviations from normal indicate that you are having trouble adapting to your training load. Baseline data is useful on a day-to-day basis as well as on a long-term basis. Significant changes in waking heart rate or waking weight over a period of two or three days necessitates immediate modification of your training, any time of the year. The intensity of your training during the Specialization Period increases the immediacy of these modifications. Long-term recording of baseline data reveals trends associated with improved fitness, such as a gradual decrease in resting heart rate due to increased cardiac stroke volume (the volume of blood pumped from the heart with each beat). The information you should record daily in the Baseline Data section of your training diary is:

Waking Heart Rate (lying down before you get out of bed)
Standing Heart Rate (Ten seconds after you get out of bed)
Waking Weight (after you use the bathroom and before you eat or
    drink)
Hours of Sleep
Quality of Sleep (restful, interrupted, tossing and turning, difficulty
    falling asleep, waking up feeling rested or still tired)
Mood (positive, motivated, discouraged, lacking motivation to train,
    stressed, lethargic)

Personal Data: Dear Diary . . .

Many athletes overlook recording Personal Data in their training diaries because they don't believe this information is relevant to training. If cycling is an integral part of your life, then your life is an integral part of your cycling. Everything going on in your professional and family life is relevant to your training, and this information needs to be included in your training diary. I have worked with athletes who were trying to figure out where their training went awry, and when I point out places where their Training and Baseline Data show signs of trouble, they interject that they were having relationship or work problems at those times as well. It is sometimes difficult to tell if the training load led to the development of the relationship problem, or if the chain of events worked the other way around, but I rarely find that the two are completely independent of each other. Stress affects you, regardless of its origin, and stress must be balanced with recovery. Record information about the stresses in your life and you will see how they affect your training. The specific data in the Personal Data section of a training diary varies from person to person, as this information is almost entirely subjective. Things to consider recording are:

Hours at work
Hours on your feet at work
Relationship status (spouse or partner)
Financial issues (Are you especially worried about money right now?)

USING YOUR TRAINING DIARY

By the time the Specialization Period begins, you have months of training information to review. The intensity of your training in the last few months leading up to your big event can contribute to diminished motivation and feelings of self-doubt. This is probably the hardest portion of the year, because you have been working hard for several months on end and there are still eight to ten weeks to go before your goal event. The quality of your training may be diminishing because you are tired physically and mentally. It is one thing to be motivated and committed to your goals when training intensity is low and you feel fresh; it is much harder to retain that motivation when your training load is high. The Specialization Period is the one last push that elevates you from pack-fodder to a fierce competitor, and athletes often have trouble keeping the difficulty of their training in perspective. As a coach, my job is to apply a training load that leads to positive adaptation. Earlier in the year, the load required was not as great, and the athlete was fresher. It was easier for the athlete to deal with training. Now the load required is immense, and the athlete has been training hard for months. Motivation starts to break down, and I have seen incredibly committed cyclists give up on workouts right in the middle of an interval because they get so frustrated. Your training diary and your coach are both critical tools to help you through the roughest portion of your training year.

The confidence-building goals you established before the season become very important now. When you are struggling during the Specialization Period, refer back to your training diary to review the things you have accomplished to this point. I sit and talk with my athletes about the fact that their physiological performance markers have steadily improved over several months. We talk about the good things they accomplished in competitions: bridging to the breakaway, winning sprints for primes, or staying in the top 15 riders through an entire race. Most important, we look at the evidence that proves that their best performances have been after periods of high training load and a regeneration week. The Specialization Period is just like any other portion of the year in that regard; the load is just higher and therefore more difficult to deal with. You have to keep things in perspective so you understand that the fatigue you are currently struggling with is part of the training process, and that you will again reap the benefits of your hard work if you stick with it until the regeneration weeks arrive. I don't believe in simply telling athletes to do what I tell them and not to ask questions. You need to understand that your training has a purpose beyond merely making you tired; that the difficulty of what you are doing will be rewarded.

When the racing season is over, you and your coach should use the information in your training diary to help establish a plan for the following season. More on that in Chapter 10.

OVERREACHING VS. OVERTRAINING

The complexity of the Specialization Period lies in the difference between overreaching and overtraining. Both relate to states of fatigue resulting from the application of intense training loads, but overreaching leads to positive adaptations and overtraining leads to negative physical and psychological effects that cause an early end to your competitive season.

Overreaching results from the application of a training load through two or more consecutive weeks of high-intensity or high-volume training. As a consequence of your training load, you may experience an increased resting heart rate and have trouble sleeping. Your heart-rate response to exercise is suppressed when you are fatigued. If you are using only heart rate to gauge intensity, this means that it takes more effort to reach a predetermined heart-rate range than when you were rested. When this is the case, your workouts will actually end up being harder than they were intended to be. This can be coupled with an increase in perceived effort for your workouts due to increased lactic-acid accumulation at submaximal workloads. Together, these factors of fatigue lead to workouts that feel more difficult than they should, even though in reality they may be harder or easier than they should be. Powermeters are very useful for determining actual workout intensity in the presence of fatigue symptoms. Your training diary also contains critical information for detecting fatigue. I consider it a problem when I see an athlete's resting heart rate increase five to ten beats and remain elevated for more than two days. Similarly, unexpected weight loss may indicate a problem with energy balance or fuel and water storage. I also look for significant variations in mood, sleep quality, and sleep hours as indications that an athlete is beginning to break down from a high training load.

The symptoms of fatigue are pronounced, but they go away after a few days of reduced training load. With overreaching, your performance improves following a one-week regeneration period. This is why I train CTS coaches to implement three weeks of training load followed by a regeneration week. Generally, two to four weeks of training is sufficient to induce an overreaching state, and the regeneration week provides the recovery time necessary for an athlete to positively adapt to the load.

Overtraining occurs when an athlete is pushed too hard and is not given enough time to adapt positively to the training load. If the training during three weeks of work is too difficult, an athlete cannot adequately recover in a week. That means the next block of training begins before the athlete has adapted fully to the previous training load. Not only will the athlete's performance suffer in the subsequent block of training, he or she will need even more time to recover and adapt afterward. When you don't allow that additional recovery time to compensate for the high training load, you are likely to end up in an overtrained state. Once overtraining sets in, the negative effects to performance are irreversible in the short term. Reversing the effects of overtraining can take between four weeks and two months, and severe cases of overtraining can take several months to recover from. Overtraining leads to a premature end to an athlete's competitive season, because it takes so long to recover enough to handle training and competition again.

The signs and symptoms of overreaching and overtraining are similar, and the mentality of committed athletes contributes to problems in differentiating one from the other. We all grew up in a society that preaches "no pain, no gain" and "more is better." Fatigue is a necessary part of the training process, and highly motivated athletes condition themselves to work through fatigue and pain. The problem is that in their zeal to improve their performance, they are the most likely population to ignore the physical and mental signs of excessive fatigue and end up in an overtrained state.

Overreaching is differentiated from overtraining by your ability to recover from a block of training in four to seven days and handle a higher training load in your next block of training. If you start a block of training after a regeneration week and you cannot perform the workouts at their prescribed intensities, you have to modify your training immediately and spend more time recovering. Alternatively, you can shorten your workouts and maintain the intensity of the shortened efforts. In either case, you are reducing your overall training load. This is a very difficult thing for athletes to handle, because they quickly become frustrated or disappointed if they have to take more time off. The overriding rule of training is that your training load has to lead to improved fitness or at least maintain a good level of fitness when compared with previous levels. If that means taking more time off than you planned for, so be it. You will be better off in the long run by taking it easy for a few days instead of pushing through more fatigue than you can handle.

I have found that committed athletes have trouble accepting the fact that overtraining is a real physical condition since it so hard to diagnose by the physiological, medical, athletic, and coaching communities. The athletes want to believe that it is all in their heads, and that they can overcome overtraining by convincing themselves that they can just deal with being tired. Experienced endurance athletes are susceptible to overtraining because they are conditioned to train through fatigue and discomfort. Inexperienced and insecure endurance athletes are susceptible to overtraining because they don't know how to recognize when they are too exhausted to train effectively. Neither group stops for the signs of overtraining, out of both insecurity and the notion that they can get an edge on the competition by training harder than everyone else. You can gain an edge on the competition by training more intelligently than everyone else, not merely by riding longer and harder. The truth is that an excessive training load leads to significant physiological consequences that negatively affect your body's ability to handle exercise at any level. I haven't found any completely reliable test to determine overtraining in an athlete, because the condition results from the interaction of many independent variables. Considered individually, none of these variables can prove that an athlete is overtrained by itself; it is the combination of conditions that indicates overtraining. Some of the mechanisms that contribute to overtraining are: central nervous system (CNS) fatigue, hormone imbalances, and glycogen depletion.

Central Nervous System Fatigue

The central nervous system (brain and spinal cord) sends electrical signals to muscle cells to tell them to contract and thereby perform work. This is an excitation process, and under normal conditions your CNS operates quickly and efficiently. Prolonged periods of excessive training cause the CNS to go into an inhibited state in order to protect itself from damage. As a result, your nerves recruit fewer muscle fibers, and the speed and strength of muscle contractions decrease. Attempting to maintain a high intensity level once your nerves are in an inhibited state requires an increase in excitation. Since the CNS also affects your emotional state, stressing it by attempting to continue to work hard leads to negative psychological effects. You become irritable, your motivation to train decreases, and you become generally discouraged. You also have trouble falling asleep, and what sleep you do get is of poor quality. CNS fatigue establishes a cycle that is difficult to get back to normal. Your poor performances reinforce your feelings of discouragement, and your lack of quality sleep contributes to continued poor training performance.

Hormone Imbalance

Excessive training also leads to hormone imbalances that negatively affect your ability to adapt to your training load. Testosterone is one of the hormones that your body uses to positively adapt to training stress. Exercise increases the amount of testosterone in your body, and testosterone has an anabolic effect: it promotes the building of muscle tissue to handle increased training loads. Exercise also causes the adrenal glands to secrete cortisol, a stressor hormone that stimulates the breakdown of protein into its building blocks, amino acids. This is a catabolic process. It is important to recovery, because tissues need amino acids to repair damage and build new cells. At appropriate levels of exercise, the catabolic effect of cortisol is balanced with the anabolic affect of testosterone to result in cellular repair and gains in muscle mass. These in turn result in improved performance.

One of the symptoms of overtraining is a disruption in the balance between cortisol and testosterone levels. Prolonged periods of hard training lead to constantly elevated levels of cortisol in the body. Normally, the onset of testosterone elevation occurs when levels of cortisol decrease. To oversimplify the matter, the catabolic effect of the cortisol makes the amino acids available, and then the testosterone levels increase so your body can use them. But if the levels of cortisol remain high, your body doesn't release enough of the testosterone it needs to complete the anabolic process. As a result, you are breaking down tissues and not rebuilding them. Over time, the damage to muscle and connective tissues (tendons and ligaments) progresses and your performance capacity decreases. It is important to note that cortisol levels increase in response to any type of stress, including emotional and lifestyle-related stress. Elevated cortisol levels have also been linked to suppression of the immune system, which makes athletes more susceptible to opportunistic infections during periods of hard training. These are the physiological reasons why the stress you experience at work or home affects your training. A highly stressed athlete may need to schedule additional recovery time between hard workouts to allow his or her body to adapt to training and prevent illness.

Glycogen Depletion

Hard exercise depletes your body's stores of glycogen. This not only affects the amount of fuel you have available for continued exercise and recovery, but it also contributes to CNS fatigue and hormone imbalances. Your body releases cortisol in response to stress, and it releases even more when you begin to run low on stored carbohydrates. Your liver can synthesize glucose from protein in a process known as gluconeogenesis. The liver needs amino acids for gluconeogenesis, and cortisol stimulates the catabolic process of liberating amino acids from tissue-bound proteins. An increase in cortisol provides the liver with the fuel it needs to create the glucose your brain and muscles need for continued activity. The CNS can utilize only glucose for fuel, so gluconeogenesis occurs primarily to supply the brain with energy. Supplying energy to muscles is a secondary concern. When you don't replenish glycogen stores by eating enough carbohydrates during exercise and immediately following exercise, you contribute to elevated levels of cortisol in the blood and an increase in the amount of protein catabolism taking place in muscle tissue. As shown earlier, elevated cortisol levels lead to immune suppression and inhibition of anabolic processes.

Your habits immediately following workouts have a large effect on your glycogen status. Uptake of glucose into muscle cells is at its highest rate and efficiency within the first 60 minutes following exercise, which is why the first hour after exercise is referred to as the "glycogen window." Exercise increases the amount of insulin in your blood, and insulin promotes the uptake of glucose from blood into muscle cells, where it is then converted to glycogen for later use. Research done by Dr. Edmund Burke, Ph.D., and others shows that ingesting protein with carbohydrates immediately following exercise further increases glucose uptake by stimulating greater insulin secretion, therefore increasing the rate of a muscle-glycogen replenishment. There has been a scientific debate about the effectiveness of using a combination of carbohydrate and protein to enhance glycogen replenishment, but the presence of protein does not hinder the rate or amount of carbohydrate absorbed into muscles. So at this point it is still a rule of thumb to use carbohydrates in conjunction with protein as an insurance policy, since there are no detrimental effects to glycogen replenishment when protein is introduced into the supplement. Dr. Burke's research suggests a 4:1 ratio of carbohydrates to protein for optimal muscle recovery, and anecdotal evidence from my athletes supports his findings.

AVOIDING OVERTRAINING

You want to avoid overtraining at all costs. It is better to arrive at an event slightly undertrained than to push so hard in training that you end up overtrained. When athletes sign up for coaching with Carmichael Training Systems, our coaches begin by determining each person's current state of fitness so we have a starting point to work from. My observations around CTS members' startup interviews are that nearly half of our athletes exhibit signs of overtraining when they come to us. I believe the prevalence of overtraining is due to the personality characteristics of endurance athletes and to a lack of understandable information available to athletes.

The most common overtraining scenario we see is the case of the "overworked executive with children." You are the people who have many obligations competing for your time, leaving only 60 to 90 minutes three to six times a week for training. You are convinced that six to nine hours of training each week is too low to be effective, so you try to compensate for low volume with high intensity. You go full-throttle from start to finish of every ride, every week. And you don't schedule regeneration weeks because you don't think you're riding enough as it is; there's no need to take even more time off. And after several months or years of this type of activity, you haven't made any gains in fitness or performance. You feel like you're wasting your time on the bike, training isn't enjoyable anymore, and you're looking for help. It may take several weeks or a few months of careful monitoring to break the overtraining cycle, but limited training time doesn't mean the end of your fitness or competitive plans. Commitment to training is not the problem; many of you will ride in the basement at 4 A.M. if that's what it takes to fit in your training. Adding structure to your program and scheduling workouts around your lifestyle lead to significant gains in your fitness and performance.

Avoiding overtraining is a matter of experience. There is no solid piece of information that alone indicates you are in an overtrained state. That's why there is so much confusion around this issue and why "overtraining" has become an overused and often misused term. If you are exhibiting the signs and symptoms that I have described in this section, I urge you to consult a coach who has experience in coaching endurance athletes. Coaches have the benefit of an objective viewpoint on your training, as well as on your physical and psychological condition. They also have experience identifying various scenarios of overtraining, so they are better equipped than most athletes to detect it.

THE ROLE OF A COACH

The Specialization Period is the time when you benefit the most from working with a good coach. A coach's role in your training goes well beyond designing your workout schedule. Your coach has to interpret your responses to training and evaluate your readiness for upcoming work. As your goal event draws closer, there's no room for mistakes or wasted training days. Training modifications need to be made swiftly and confidently so that you, as the athlete, can maintain your focus on your event instead of worrying about how many intervals you should do today.

My phone rings off the hook during the summer months when the majority of my athletes are in their Specialization Periods, and I am not alone. All the coaches at CTS put in long hours monitoring their athletes' training progress and watching for signs of fatigue and overtraining. It is your job to train and rest, and it's our job to tell you when and how to train and rest.

In order to do the best job for you, your coach needs to hear from you frequently. I tell athletes I work with that I want to know everything they would tell a doctor. I need to know about the little aches and pains, the rashes, the runny nose, and the diarrhea. I also need to know about the great set of intervals, the awesome performance in a training criterium, and the restful nights of sleep. Don't tell me you "feel fine." The question "How are you?" should trigger a flood of information coming my way. This is true throughout the year, but it is absolutely critical during the Specialization Period. Earlier I talked about the difficulty of differentiating overreaching from overtraining. The more information you provide, the better I can tailor your training and make sure you are overreaching and getting enough rest to avoid overtraining.

Clarity and Consistency

There is no time for uncertainty in training prescription during the Specialization Period. Athletes who don't work with coaches often question their training programs during this time of year because the workouts are difficult and fatigue affects their mental outlook. This causes increased anxiety about their readiness for competition and often leads to unnecessary or incorrect modifications to training. Your coach is in a much better position to maintain an objective viewpoint on the appropriateness of your workouts. Believe in your coach and keep the lines of communication open when you are fatigued and lack confidence in your training program.

Avoid the urge to test your strength and power too many times during the Specialization Period. You are feeling strong and fast during this period, and it is very tempting to hit the throttle and show yourself and everyone else how strong you are. Testing yourself on training rides weeks before your event inadvertently increases your training load and causes you to reach peak fitness too early. It also decreases the length of time you can maintain peak conditioning. Follow your coach's program. Race-intensity efforts, training races, and competitions should all be part of your program during the Specialization Period. Save your energy for those events, and have fun breaking people's legs at those times. In between those workouts and competitions, stick to the intensities your coach prescribes.

Sounding Board

As a competitive athlete, you have to be wary about your interactions with teammates, managers, and even family members. Discuss your frustrations about team situations, travel problems, or family disturbances with your coach before others, only because increased stress and anxiety often lead to poor communication decisions. Your coach understands the effect of training and competition on the rest of your life and can help you deal with sport-related issues without alienating or angering the people around you.

Talk with your coach about tactical race plans and backup plans around travel, accommodations, warmup, and racing. These things are all parts of being completely prepared for your event, and you can benefit from your coach's experience to avoid pitfalls and mistakes you would otherwise never know about. For instance, are you prepared for the airline to lose your bike? If you have your shoes, pedals, and helmet in your carry-on, you can most likely finagle a bike to race on. If your shoes and pedals are with the bike, it will be much more difficult to find the equipment you need for competition.

Don't be afraid to tell your coach that you are worried, anxious, nervous, or scared. Being brave for your coach is not helpful to your success. Younger and less-experienced athletes often try to impress their coaches with the workload they can handle. This was especially true with the U.S. National Team in the early 1990s. Those guys (including George Hincapie, Lance Armstrong, Kevin Livingston, and Bobby Julich) would not openly admit they were tired, no matter what signs of exhaustion they were exhibiting. To them, admitting you were tired was admitting you were weaker than the guy next to you. It took a while, but once they stopped trying to prove how strong they were, they started making significant performance gains. Be honest with your coach so he or she has accurate information to use when designing your program. You may not want to let the competition know you're worried about the long climb in next week's race, or that you get scared cornering at high speeds, but don't be afraid to tell your coach. It is his job to help you deal with issues that are keeping you from succeeding as an athlete, and he won't think any less of you because you don't feel particularly comfortable bumping handlebars at 40 mph in the middle of a corner.

THE KEYS TO A SUCCESSFUL SPECIALIZATION PERIOD

1. Use a field test and competitive performances to make sure you have the aerobic engine and lactate-threshold conditioning to handle the increase in workload from the Preparation Period.
2. Prepare yourself for the effects of hard training. Recognize that your motivation may suffer due to fatigue, but that the fatigue is a temporary and necessary component of training. Maintain perspective and have confidence that your hard work will reap huge benefits.
3. Monitor your training carefully. Use your training diary to watch for significant and lasting variations in resting heart rate, waking weight, power output, and heart rate response to exercise. The faster you recognize the signs of overreaching and overtraining, the better chance you have of promoting overreaching and preventing overtraining.

4. Talk with a coach. The Specialization Period is the hardest training period of the year, and there is no room for mistakes. You have worked hard for several months to get to this part of the year; don't let fatigue-induced poor decisions ruin everything you accomplished.

SPECIALIZATION PERIOD TRAINING EXAMPLES

The Specialization Period is very intense and extremely dependent on the work you have done to get to this point of the year. HighSpeedSprints develop power, and starting the sprint from high speed develops your coordination and bike-handling skills. Other workouts, like PowerIntervals and DescendingIntervals, play large roles in your ability to repeat maximum efforts. Both of these workouts feature short, highly intense efforts with very little recovery time between them. The time between intervals is too short for you to completely recover before starting the next one, and the lack of recovery is critical to the workout's success.

Pay careful attention to details concerning your recovery and nutrition during this time, because it is very easy to fall behind on either rest or fuel when you are training so hard. The Specialization Period can be mentally and emotionally taxing as well, but remember that there is light at the end of the tunnel. The weeks leading up to your goal event are the peaking process, where rest and regeneration will help you rebound to new heights of performance.

Specialization Period Training Examples

	MONDAY	TUESDAY	WEDNESDAY	
Intermediate 4-Day				
Week 1	Rest Day	2hr EM w/5x3min PI	1hr EM	
Week 2	Rest Day	2hr EM w/6x3min PI	1.25hr EM	
Week 3	Rest Day	2hr EM w/75/60/45/ 30sec x 2 sets DI	1.5hr FM	
Week 4	Rest Day	1hr RR	1.5hr FM	
Advanced 4-Day				
Week 1	Rest Day	2hr EM w/6x3min MT	1hr EM	
Week 2	Rest Day	2hr EM w/7x3min MT	1.25hr EM	
Week 3	Rest Day	2hr EM w/75/60/45/ 30sec x 3 sets DI	2hr EM w/75/60/45/ 30sec x 2 sets DI	
Week 4	Rest Day	1.5hr RR	2hr EM	
Intermediate 6-Day				
Week 1	Rest Day	2hr EM w/5x3min PI	1hr EM	
Week 2	Rest Day	2hr EM w/6x3min PI	1.25hr EM	
Week 3	Rest Day	2hr EM w/75/60/45/ 30sec x 2 sets DI	1.5hr EM	
Week 4	Rest Day	1hr RR	1.5hr EM	
Advanced 6-Day				
Week 1	Rest Day	2hr EM w/6x3min PI	1hr EM	
Week 2	Rest Day	2hr EM w/7x3min PI	1.25hr EM	
Week 3	Rest Day	2hr EM w/75/60/45 30sec x 3 sets DI	2hr EM w/75/60/45/ 30sec x 2 sets DI	
Week 4	Rest Day	1.5hr RR	2hr EM	

	THURSDAY	FRIDAY	SATURDAY	SUNDAY
	2hr EM w/5x10sec HSS	Rest Day	2.5hr EM w/40min RS	2hr EM
	2hr EM w/5x3min PI	Rest Day	2.25hr EM w/45min RS	2.75hr EM
	2hr EM w/75/60/45/ 30sec 1 set DI	Rest Day	3hr EM	2.5hr EM w/6x10sec HSS
	2hr EM w/8min under, 2 min over x 3 OU	Rest Day	2.5hr EM	2.5hr EM w/45min RS
	2hr EM w/6x3min PI	Rest Day	2.5hr EM w/60min RS	2hr EM
	2hr EM w/8x10sec HSS	Rest Day	2.5hr EM w/75min RS	2.75hr EM
	1.5hr EM	Rest Day	3hr EM	2.5hr EM w/8x10sec HSS
	2hr EM w/8min under, 2min over x 4 OU	Rest Day	2.5hr EM	3hr EM w/45min RS
	2hr EM w/5x10sec HSS	45min RR	2.5hr EM w/40min RS	2hr EM
	2hr EM w/5x3min PI	1hr RR	2.25hr EM w/45min RS	2.75hr EM
	2hr EM w/75/60/45/ 30sec x 1 set DI	1hr RR	3hr EM	2.5hr EM w/6x10sec HSS
	2hr EM w/8min under, 2min over x 3 OU	1hr RR	2.5hr EM	2.5hr EM w/45min RS
	2hr EM w/6x3min PI	1hr RR	2.5hr EM w/60min RS	2hr EM
	2hr EM w/8x10sec HSS	1.25hr RR	2.5hr EM w/75min RS	2.75hr EM
	1.5hr EM	1.25hr RR	3hr EM	2.5hr EM w/8x10sec HSS
	2hr EM w/8min under, 2min over x 4 OU	1hr RR	2.5hr EM	3hr EM w/45min RS

9

Peaking: One More Step to Go

T HE PROCESS OF PEAKING for an event refreshes the mind and the body. In the last four weeks leading up to your goal event, your overall fitness doesn't change drastically. The work you have done over the past several months has enhanced your aerobic engine, increased your sustainable power, and improved your racing ability. The last step en route to your ultimate ride is a short period of unloading and supercompensation.

Peaking for an event involves short, high-intensity workouts, full recovery between sessions, and impeccable timing. The intensity of training and the importance of recovery are similar to the Specialization Period; in fact, peaking is really just an extension of the Specialization Period. Timing becomes critical because you have to determine the best time to reduce training load in order to elevate performance to its highest level of the year.

I usually apply training loads in four-week macrocycles (four one-week microcycles), with three weeks of gradually increasing training intensity and volume followed by one week of regeneration. The next macrocycle begins at a training load 10 to 15 percent higher than that of the previous one, and the regeneration week is what makes the increase in training load possible. During that week, your body takes advantage of the reduced stress to repair itself, build new tissues, and generally adapt in anticipation of future stresses. The Peaking Process follows a similar premise, but on a larger scale. One week is sufficient to adapt and reap the benefits of three weeks of training, but it takes several weeks to achieve the same effect from several months of accumulated training. In some ways, you can

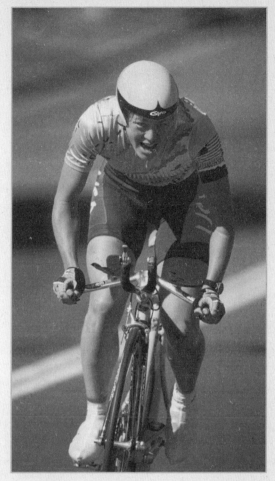

Mari Holden's peaking process in 2000 netted her an Olympic Silver Medal, and a World Championship a few weeks later. *Photo © by Graham Watson*

think of the peaking process as an extended regeneration week that enables you to reap the benefits of your entire training program.

Timing becomes critical during the Peaking Process because you have to weigh the benefits of recovery and regeneration carefully with the risk of becoming stale and losing aerobic fitness. Upon initially reducing your training load, your level of fatigue decreases as you replenish glycogen stores and adapt to the previous stress. There is a supercompensation effect that elevates your performance capacity to a level above where it was before the most recent application of training stress. This supercompensation effect is relatively short-lived, and if you reduce your training load and volume too early before your big event, the effect goes away before your can use it to your advantage. On the other hand, if you wait too long before reducing the training load, you are not leaving enough time to replenish and regenerate and you won't reach supercompensation in time for your event.

The method for reducing training load during your peaking process should be through reducing volume and frequency but not intensity. Your schedule should include shorter rides and fewer workouts per week, but the workouts in your schedule should be very intense. The duration of the peaking process is shorter for stage-race competitors (approximately 1.5 to 2.5 weeks) and longer for criterium and time-trial competitors (3 to 4 weeks). As I discussed in Chapter 6, it is more important for one-day racers to be as fresh and rested as possible for their events, while the stage racers need to preserve as much aerobic conditioning as possible.

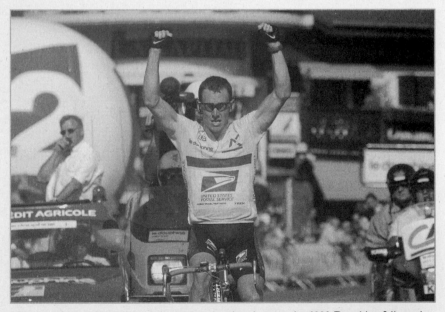

Some said Lance Armstrong peaked too early when he won the 2002 Dauphine Libere, but I've always said it's better to be ready early than too late. *Photo © by Graham Watson*

As I have said several times already, it is better to reach complete preparation too early as opposed to too late. There is no way to drastically increase the rate of regeneration to compensate for a lack of recovery time. There is, however, a way to extend the duration of peak performance capacity through "feathering" training and recovery over a period of a few weeks. This involves using short, high-intensity efforts and periods of full recovery. You don't want your training efforts to induce heavy fatigue, but you do want the efforts to be hard enough to maintain a high level of competitive readiness. Keep in mind that you are not significantly adding to your fitness in the final few weeks leading up to your event; you are only affecting how much of your accumulated fitness you can access.

Try thinking of the peaking process in this way: the pressure of the Specialization Period compressed the elements of your fitness into a valuable and brilliant gem, and peaking is the process of mining and polishing that gem. You developed a diamond through months of training and work, and the finished product is hidden beneath layers of fatigue. During the peaking process, your goal is to strip away the fatigue in order to reveal the diamond in all of its luster.

TRAINING IN THE PEAKING PROCESS

During the peaking process, your training revolves primarily around short efforts at and above race-intensity. Through the Foundation and Preparation Periods, blocks of training were focused on improving specific energy systems. During the Specialization Period, your workouts tapped into all of your energy systems and improved the efficiency with which you integrated them all together. Now the workouts are similar, but the speed and acceleration increase. Workouts like PowerIntervals, SpeedIntervals, and HighSpeedSprints provide short bursts of stimulus to all of your energy systems, helping you adapt to the rapid changes in effort that are found in competition.

When the peaking process is proceeding as it should, athletes react quickly during workouts, and they recover very quickly from hard efforts. It is as if their energy systems have adopted an agility normally reserved for gymnasts and acrobats. If an athlete tells me she felt sluggish at the beginning of intervals during her workout, and that her heart rate and breathing were slow to respond to the sudden increase in intensity, I take the information as a sign of fatigue. The same is true if it takes more than three or four minutes for her heart rate and breathing rate to return to normal aerobic levels after maximal efforts. It is important for the athlete to tell me about this immediately following the workout so I can determine whether the following day's workout needs to be modified. By carefully monitoring training during the peaking process, she can apply enough training stress to maintain high performance, but not enough to make her tired.

Training is like an On/Off switch during this period. When you are on your bike, you're On. The efforts are quick, hard, and powerful. When you are off the bike, and during recovery rides as well, you are Off. There should be no training stimulus outside of the specified workouts, only recovery. Active recovery is still more beneficial than complete rest, so I recommend light spins around the neighborhood instead of just lounging on the couch. However, you should spend as much time as you can on the couch when you are not on the bike. Just because your training volume has decreased, this is not the time to embark on major landscaping projects. When you are training, you need to give it your full attention and effort. When you are not training, you need to do as little as possible. There is an old saying, and I don't know its origin, but it goes something like this: "Why stand when you could sit? Why sit when you could lie down? Why walk when you could ride?"

Of course, it is not realistic for most of us to put life on hold for a few weeks while peaking for an event. The grass still needs mowing and your boss and family still need attention. But even slight modifications to your normal schedule and habits can increase the effectiveness of your peaking process. Get a little more rest by going to bed 30 to 60 minutes earlier than usual. Plan meals in advance to ensure that your diet includes good sources of complex carbohydrates and protein. Avoid junk food and lay off the beer for a few weeks (save it to celebrate your great performance). If you normally get massages, schedule a few extra sessions in the weeks before your event. If you don't normally get massages, don't start now. This is not the time to experiment with anything new, and that includes new equipment, position changes, and nutritional supplements.

The benefits of peaking are somewhat short-lived because your aerobic conditioning suffers while you are focusing on race-intensity work. The training rides during the peaking process are too short and too difficult to provide much training benefit to the aerobic system. This is why peaking too early is a problem. Most athletes can't maintain optimal race-fitness longer than three to five weeks before their aerobic endurance begins to break down. More experienced athletes can extend this period to five to seven weeks through several years of consistent training.

Once your aerobic system starts to weaken, the number of hard efforts you can handle and recover from decreases. Rapidly losing power in the middle of a criterium is one strong indication of this problem. You had enough energy and power to race aggressively and normally for a while, but then your power disappeared and you were toast. And this happened after a normal warmup and despite the fact you had enough food and water in you to easily make it through the whole race. In this case, your race-specific fitness (peak power, repeatability, etc.) isn't the problem. The problem is that your aerobic foundation is eroding underneath you and it can no longer contribute as much energy. That means your anaerobic system is contributing a higher percentage of your overall energy output. Unfortunately, it's burning fuel far faster than your aerobic system did and producing lactic acid faster than you can clear it. This scenario is extremely frustrating, but resist the urge to continue racing in hopes of "just one more good day." The longer you wait to give your aerobic system the boost it needs, the more it erodes. When you catch it quickly, one or two weeks of endurance training (Tempo workouts, long endurance rides) is all it takes to get back to top form.

NUTRITIONAL CONSIDERATIONS

Many athletes have the urge to lose weight during the Specialization Period and peaking process. They want to increase their power-to-weight ratios, and figure their training improved the power portion of the equation and their diet can improve the weight portion. While that is true, this is not the best time of year to lose weight. Weight loss is the result of expending more calories than you ingest by about 500 or more calories per day. Right now, your body needs fuel for recovery and replenishment, and purposely inducing a significant caloric deficit is contrary to your goal of recovery for quality training. Additionally, trying to lose weight can confuse issues around overtraining. Remember, weight loss is one of the symptoms indicative of overtraining. If you are on the borderline between overreaching and overtraining anyway, how will you know if your weight loss is a good thing? A caloric deficit during the Specialization Period and peaking process tends to decrease the quality of your training because of chronic glycogen depletion, decreased recovery, and increased susceptibility to infections.

Ideally, your caloric intake and expenditure are nearly equal while you are training. Your goal is to provide the nutrients your body needs to recover and adapt to your training load. During the Specialization Period and peaking process, your training is race-specific and so is your nutrition. Just as you cut out extraneous workouts and energy expenditures, cut out foods that don't enhance your ability to train and compete optimally. Replace colas with more water, and junk food snacks with more fruits and vegetables. You can even take a look at the quality of the ingredients you use in cooking. Seek breads and pastas with a higher percentage of complex carbohydrates (multi-grain bread instead of white bread), fresh fish, leaner cuts of meat and chicken, and fewer processed foods. Your grocery bill may increase a bit, but finding higher-quality sources of carbohydrate, protein, fish oils, and monounsaturated fats is worth the extra cost. Better fuel burns hotter and cleaner.

Supplements should be used sparingly throughout the year. I would rather see athletes obtain as much of their nutrition as possible from natural foods as opposed to powders and pills. Supplements should be just that, nutrients added to your diet to ensure that you obtain what you need. For the majority of amateur athletes, I believe a good multivitamin with antioxidants is a good idea as a nutritional insurance policy. With the exception of the fat-soluble vitamins A, D, E, and K, your body will simply excrete vitamins and minerals it already has enough of.

As I've mentioned, large concentrations of fat-soluble vitamins and iron can be toxic. Before you start loading up on vitamins, it is best to be aware of the amounts of these nutrients already found in your diet. A nutrition professional can determine the current nutrient balance of your diet and help you correct deficiencies and optimize intake.

Over the years, people have talked a lot about Lance Armstrong's Tour de France weight and his eating practices in the months beforehand. It is true that Lance's diet is extremely regimented during the Specialization Period in

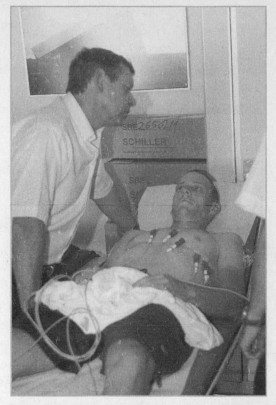

Lance Armstrong at the required medical tests prior to the Tour de France. He is extremely lean at his 72-kg race weight, and he only maintains this weight for a few weeks. *Photo © by Graham Watson*

order to bring his weight down to around 72 kgs (158 lbs) by the Tour de France. It is important to understand that what Lance does is an extreme case, because the Tour de France is an extreme event. I don't recommend that any other athletes I work with attempt the same level of dietary restriction. There is a substantial risk of losing power and training capacity through restricting caloric intake. There can also be a negative effect on the rate and effectiveness of recovery. Overall, I believe that for most people the benefits of being healthier and more powerful override the benefit of being one or two kilograms (two to five pounds) lighter.

THE PSYCHOLOGY OF PEAKING

Having more time on your hands is one consequence of reducing your training load, and it can help you or hurt you. On one hand, you have time to relax, visualize a great race, and double-check all your equipment, accommodations, and travel plans. On the other hand, you have plenty of time to worry about your preparation, your plans, and your performance. I have found good preparation and appropriate goals to be very effective in reducing pre-race anxiety during the peaking process. When you can review your training and clearly recognize the progression of your fitness and racing skills, it is easier to logically dispel doubts about your readiness to compete.

The reduction in training volume also triggers anxiety in some athletes because they erroneously believe their fitness will disappear. It is much harder to improve fitness than to lose it, and you wouldn't lose any appreciable power or capacity if you took an entire week of complete rest. Plus, detraining affects you from the top down. Your race-specific fitness would go first (peak power, VO_2, repeatability, agility), followed by your LT power (sustainable power at threshold), and finally your aerobic system. Even though the overall volume of your training is reduced during the peaking process, the intensity and specificity of the workouts ensures the maintenance of your race-fitness. The short duration of the peaking process reduces the chances or degree of aerobic-system degradation.

Athletes who are confident with their preparation and fitness can still suffer from anxiety in the weeks leading up to their event. Performance anxiety is normal, but if unchecked, it can be disastrous. It is good to be a little anxious about your goal event because you will probably be more attentive to details regarding nutrition, equipment, rest, and transportation. But too much anxiety regarding competition leads to trouble sleeping and eating, either of which is enough to negatively affect your performance. Remember to focus on the things you can control: your preparation, warmup, nutrition, rest, and tactics. Look to your previous race experiences for confidence in your ability to handle your bike, race aggressively, and control your destiny.

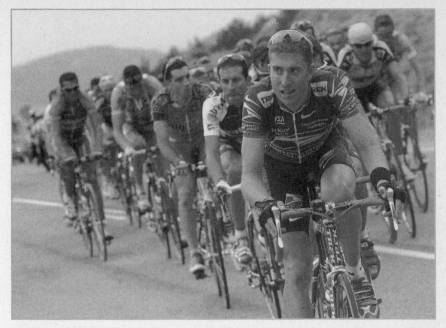

Christian VandeVelde leading the pack on the Sierra Nevada climb of the 2002 Tour of Spain. His peaking process made him one of team-leader Roberto Heras's most valuable assets. *Photo © by Graham Watson*

ILLNESS, INJURIES, BURNOUT

The downside to being a committed athlete is often your "ability" to forge ahead with training in the face of fatigue, aches, and pains. Many athletes see their stories of training through illnesses and injuries as badges of courage. They are inspired by professional athletes who return to competition within days of suffering serious injuries, of football players who valiantly play on in spite of broken bones and torn ligaments. Often, the prevailing belief is that the strongest athletes are the ones who don't let anything stand in their way. What you are forgetting is that professional athletes are paid to take serious risks with their health and well-being, and they eventually pay huge prices for the decisions of their youth. Illness, pain, and burnout are your body's way of slowing you down before you can inflict more serious damage. It is important to listen to your body and respond appropriately so you can continue enjoying cycling as a senior citizen.

Illness

The onset of opportunistic illnesses, nagging injuries, and feelings of burnout are signs that you may have tried to stretch a peak too far. Opportunistic illnesses are things like upper-respiratory infections, colds, sore throats, and stomach bugs. The germs that cause these ailments are around all the time, but your immune system is normally strong enough to beat them. When you are exhausted, your body doesn't have enough fuel to both repair tissues and adequately power your immune system. Elevated levels of cortisol (see Chapter 7 for more on cortisol) also lead to suppression of the immune system, allowing a normally defeatable bug to infect you.

The safest course of action is to take some time off from training when you are sick. For the most part, your fitness will be less affected by a few days off than by training with symptoms and making the illness worse. But since experience has proven that athletes abhor the thought of skipping workouts unless they are bedridden, here are a few guidelines you should follow regarding training and illness:

1. If your symptoms are restricted to your neck and head (runny nose, scratchy throat, sinus congestion), reduce your training volume and intensity and start your ride. If you feel miserable within the first 20 minutes of the ride, turn around and go home. If you feel well enough to continue the ride, keep the ride under two hours, and I don't recommend performing LT-intensity intervals or anything harder.
2. If your symptoms are in your chest or are accompanied by achy joints, vomiting, or fever, don't even get dressed to ride. These symptoms are often associated with viruses affecting your whole body, and training will only make the situation worse. In the most extreme cases, intense exercise can lead to a viral infection of the heart, which can be fatal.
3. Return to light and moderate training when your symptoms lessen significantly. You don't necessarily have to wait until all symptoms disappear completely, as chest and sinus congestion sometimes linger for several days after the other symptoms of ill-

ness are gone. Restrict yourself to aerobic-intensity training for twice as long as you were sick. For example, if your cold lasted one week, you shouldn't resume LT workouts for two weeks after your symptoms have cleared up.

4. Once your period of aerobic training is completed, avoid the mistake of trying to compensate for missed training by drastically increasing volume or intensity. This is a common tendency and has consistent results: you will get sick again in a few weeks. A short illness (less than ten days) will not seriously affect your ability to be prepared for your goal event. However, repeated illnesses totaling three weeks of missed training will hurt your progress.

Injuries

During a long cycling season, it is common for athletes to develop small aches and pains. Maybe your knee aches a little from time to time, or your shoulder still hurts from last month's crash. The important dis-

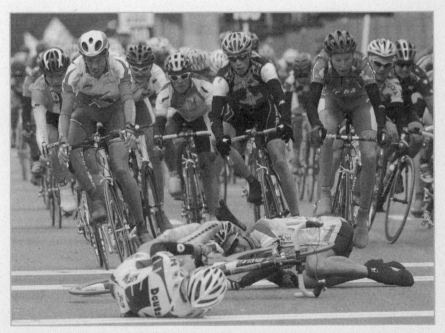

Crashes are an unfortunate but inevitable part of bike racing. Take care of yourself so small injuries don't become bigger problems. *Photo © by Graham Watson*

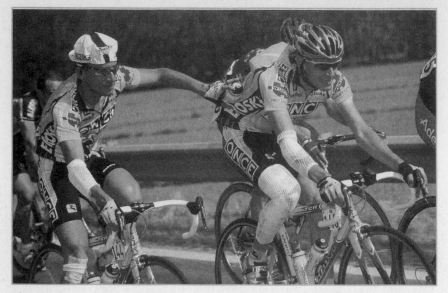

Members of the ONCE team demonstrating proper treatment for road rash.
Photo © by Graham Watson

tinction to make is whether the injury is continually getting better (healing) or worse. If pain persists at the same level or worsens over a three-to-four-day period, take a few days off from training. If the pain is still present when you resume training, see a physician. In the case of crash-related injuries, get medical clearance to continue to train and compete. What you perceive as a sore shoulder may in fact be a separated shoulder with significant soft-tissue damage. Soreness and abrasions take a while to heal, and you can generally continue training unless the injury hinders your ability to control your bike safely.

Continuing to race and train hard through small injuries only makes them worse, and since most amateur athletes can only afford medical care for acute injuries and crashes, small injuries tend to get bigger before they get treated. Many of the aches and pains you can't pinpoint to one moment of onset are due to problems with bike fit or flexibility. Increased volume or intensity of racing and training increases your susceptibility to these types of injuries. Refer back to Chapter 6 for information on bike fit, and Chapter 5 for information on stretching in order to prevent injury.

Treatment of Road Rash Unfortunately, road rash is a fact of life for competitive cyclists. If you are on your bike 280 days a year, chances are pretty good that you will fall off of it a few times. After crashing more times than I'd like to remember, I can give you this good method for treating your abrasions*:

1. After checking to make sure you aren't more seriously injured or at risk of being hit by a car or another cyclist, use a water bottle to rinse the affected area. This helps you determine how serious the wound is and reduces the amount of debris stuck to you.

2. When you get home from the ride, or back to your car after a race (you should always carry a first-aid kit in your race bag), thoroughly wash the area with soap and water. As much as you don't want to do this, you are going to have to scrub the wound a bit to get the grit, sand, and debris out of it. If you can do this within about 15 minutes of the crash, it won't hurt quite as much. Endorphins, your natural painkillers, are pumped into your bloodstream in response to the trauma of crashing. For a short period of time, you can clean your wounds without as much pain.

3. After you rinse the soap off, inspect the abrasion and look for larger pieces of debris, small stones, glass, etc. It is alright to remove small rocks and debris from the wound, but do not remove any object that has impaled you (sticks, nails, etc.). If you have been impaled like this, loosely bandage the wound and seek medical attention immediately.

4. It is best to keep abrasions moist throughout the healing process. Scabs are convenient, but they lead to increased healing time and scarring. Keeping the wound moist with antibiotic ointments retains the elasticity of your skin as it heals, and thus reduces the stiffness and soreness associated with movement. This is especially true around joints. Apply a thin coat of ointment to a bandage and cover the abrasion.

*These recommendations adhere to Red Cross guidelines for treatment of skin abrasions, and I recommend consulting a health-care professional for evaluation and treatment after crashes, even seemingly minor ones.

5. Change your bandages frequently, at least twice a day in the first few days following the crash. Wash the abrasion with soap and water each time you change the bandages, and continue to use antibiotic ointment. The netting you see holding bandages over professional cyclists' limbs is available through medical-supply houses, and if you have trouble finding it, sections of women's stockings work well too (and come in more styles and colors).

   You will probably notice how much dirt and debris is present the first time you change your bandages. Your body knows the difference between foreign objects and things that are parts of you. By keeping the wound moist and bandaging it, you are helping your body push out small foreign objects that could otherwise lead to infections.

6. Stop bandaging only when there is no longer any seepage from the wound, and when new skin has completely formed over the area. This new skin is very susceptible to sunburn, so take special care to generously apply sunscreen to it. Vitamin-E ointments are also helpful for reducing scarring. If at any time during the healing process the seepage from the wound is discolored, foul-smelling, or chunky, the wound may be infected and you should seek medical attention. Fever, and swelling and redness around the edges of the wound, are also signs of infection.

During periods of heavier training and racing, wounds may take longer to heal. Growing new skin takes a lot of energy, and if you are already struggling to get enough energy for recovery, there may not be much left for building skin cells. Abrasions that don't seem to heal are a sign that you are at risk for fatigue-related problems, including overtraining and illness. When you are exhausted, small aches and pains linger longer than they should, if they go away at all, because you don't have the fuel to repair the damage.

Burnout

Burnout is common among athletes with lofty racing goals and long seasons. The high emotional commitment to training and racing takes its toll, and you eventually become frustrated simply with being committed. Training starts to feel like work—like one more thing you have to do before the day is over. Your excitement around racing disappears and your performance suffers as a result. Burnout differs from overtraining in that it is a mental phenomenon that leads to diminished will to perform, whereas overtraining is a physiological condition that consequently leads to frustration and reduced motivation.

In an ironic twist, the emotional strain that leads to burnout is highest during the weeks before the event you have been principally training for. I have worked with athletes who wanted to quit the sport completely three weeks before the best performances of their careers. Emotionally, they'd had enough of the regimented training, the focus on their diet, and the commitment of getting on their bikes each day. At times I had to talk them into training because I knew the long-term effect of letting them quit would be disastrous. Training is difficult, and every athlete is tempted to quit or skip intervals when no one else is looking. As a coach, it is my job to push an athlete when it is appropriate and rein him in when it is necessary, and to do either with only the athlete's best interest at heart.

You can avoid burnout by planning breaks in your training and racing schedule. These breaks are separate from regeneration weeks or the Transition Period. I'm talking about vacations from competition and regimented training. The first type of vacation is simply time off the bike. Put your bike away and head to a warm beach for ten days in June. Sure, you're going to miss a few criteriums, but if your goal event is in September, the time off is necessary to recharge your desire and commitment to training. By the time you get home, you'll be fired up to train again. More important, you will still have the desire to train in August. The second type of vacation is on your bike, but has nothing to do with regimented training or specific workouts. Schedule a short bike trip during a period of aerobic endurance training and go somewhere new. Many of the cyclists living in Colorado take trips south to Arizona a few times in the winter. The riding and the weather are nice, and the change of scenery helps them to retain motivation.

Cycling camps are another way of keeping yourself motivated to train. Prior to going to camp, a desire to be in decent shape to enjoy the camp motivates many athletes to train. And then the camp itself is a new

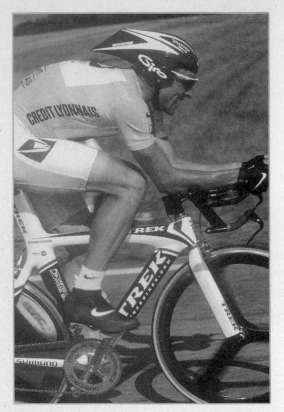

Lance Armstrong during the final time trial of the 2000 Tour de France. He gains more power each time he completes a peaking process. *Photo © by Graham Watson*

cycling experience that improves your training habits and handling skills. The positive training environment and people you meet at a cycling camp continue to affect you long after you return home. Some cycling camps focus on training, while others are designed around sightseeing or watching great cycling events like the Tour de France, the Tour of Italy, or the Tour of Spain. I attend most of the camps that Carmichael Training Systems hosts during the year, and I believe camps can be effectively used to enhance your training for a competitive goal, and alternatively, that good performance during a camp can be the goal your training prepares you for.

WRAPPING UP THE PEAKING PROCESS

Executed properly, peaking can increase your performance capacity by up to about 15 percent. This gives you a distinct advantage over athletes who either train right up to an event or think of peaking as a cessation of training in the final week before competing. Keep good records of your training activities and your subjective thoughts on how you feel in the weeks leading up to your event. This information will be extremely useful in planning for subsequent peaking processes, either within the same cycling season or for the following year. Lance Armstrong's peaking process has undergone significant refinements over the past several years, and as a result I believe he has been stronger at the beginning of every Tour de France since 1999.

PEAKING PROCESS
TRAINING EXAMPLES

Hard efforts and a lot of rest characterize training during the peaking process. The efforts are designed to maintain your agility on the bike as well as your ability to rapidly respond to changes in intensity. Your workouts should not be long enough to induce significant fatigue, because the other main goal of the peaking process is to deliver you to the start line rested and fresh.

Peaking Process Training Examples

	MONDAY	TUESDAY	WEDNESDAY	
Intermediate 5-Day				
Week 1	Rest Day	2hr EM w/4x30sec x 2 sets SI	1hr EM	
Week 2	Rest Day	2hr EM w/5x30sec x 2 sets SI	1.25hr EM	
Week 3	Rest Day	2hr EM w/8min under, 3min over x 3 OU	1hr EM	
Week 4	Rest Day	1.5hr EM	2hr EM w/75/60/45 30sec x 1 set DI	
Advanced 5-Day				
Week 1	Rest Day	2hr EM w/6x30sec x 2 sets SI	1hr EM	
Week 2	Rest Day	2hr EM w/7x30sec x 2 sets SI	2hr EM w/6x30sec x 2 sets SI	
Week 3	Rest Day	2hr EM w/8min under, 3min over x 4 OU	1hr EM	
Week 4	Rest Day	1.5hr EM	2hr EM w/75/60/45 30sec x 2 sets DI	
Intermediate 6-Day				
Week 1	Rest Day	2hr EM w/4x30sec x 2 sets SI	1hr EM	
Week 2	Rest Day	2hr EM w/5x30sec x 2 sets SI	1.25hr EM	
Week 3	Rest Day	2hr EM w/8min under, 3min over x 3 OU	1hr EM	
Week 4	Rest Day	1.5 hr EM	2hr EM w/75/60/45/ 30sec x 1 set DI	
Advanced 6-Day				
Week 1	Rest Day	2hr EM w/6x30sec x 2 sets SI	1hr EM	
Week 2	Rest Day	2hr EM w/7x30sec x 2 sets SI	2hr EM w/6x30sec x 2 sets SI	
Week 3	Rest Day	2hr EM w/8min under, 3min over x 4 OU	1hr EM	
Week 4	Rest Day	1.5hr EM	2hr EM w/75/60/45 30sec x 2 sets DI	

	THURSDAY	FRIDAY	SATURDAY	SUNDAY
	2hr EM w/4x30sec x 2 sets SI	Rest Day	2hr EM	2.5hr EM w/6x10sec HSS
	2hr EM w/8min under, 2min over x 3 OU	Rest Day	2.25hr EM w/45min RS	2hr EM
	1hr EM	Rest Day	2hr EM	1hr RR
	1.25hr EM	Rest Day	1hr EM w/2x2min PI	Event
	2hr EM w/6x30sec x 2 sets SI	Rest Day	2hr EM	2.5hr EM w/8x10sec HSS
	1.25 hr EM	Rest Day	2.25hr EM w/60min RS	2hr EM
	1.5hr EM	Rest Day	2hr EM	1hr RR
	1.25hr EM	Rest Day	1.5hr EM w/3x2min PI	Event
	2hr EM w/4x30sec x 2 sets SI	45min RM	2hr EM	2.5hr EM w/6x10sec HSS
	2hr EM w/8min under, 2min over x 3 OU	1hr RM	2.25hr EM w/45min RS	2hr EM
	1hr EM	1hr RM	2hr EM	1hr RR
	1.25hr EM	1hr RM	1hr EM w/2x2min PI	Event
	2hr EM w/6x30sec x 2 sets SI	1hr RM	2hr EM	2.5hr EM w/8x10sec HSS
	1.25hr EM	1.25hr RM	2.25hr EM w/60min RS	2hr EM
	1.5hr EM	1.25hr RM	2hr EM	1hr RR
	1.25hr EM	1hr RM	1.5hr EM w/3x2min PI	Event

10

The 100% Ready Athlete

ALL OF YOUR WORK and planning culminate in the emergence of the 100% Ready Athlete. At this point everything comes together and your mental, physical, and emotional states are at the pinnacle of competitive readiness. You are excited and motivated to race, confident in your abilities to compete at your best, and in the best physical condition of the year. Revel in your strength, be proud of it, and let everyone see it; this is your reward for the months of work.

THE CHARACTER OF THE 100% READY ATHLETE

Everything just "clicks" when you are completely ready for competition. Your body responds immediately to requests to either speed up or slow down. It feels like you have unfettered access to every ounce of your power at all times. No matter how hard you push, it's as if you're just floating on the pedals. Your awareness and coordination are perfect; the most complicated movements on the bike are effortless and require no conscious thought. You're calm in regard to nervousness and anxiety, but excited regarding the opportunity to compete. All of this combines to provide happiness and confidence in yourself. The 100% Ready Athlete is calm and happy, with the gleam of determination and confidence in his or her eyes.

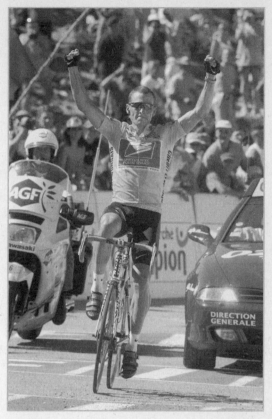

Lance Armstrong at the Tour de France is the epitome of the 100% Ready Athlete. *Photo © by Graham Watson*

Competitive Arousal

Competitive arousal has nothing to do with Viagra; it refers to your level of excitement in the hours before your event. Your brain and body cannot be separated, and both have to be charged to the right level in order for you to compete at your best. Everyone experiences different degrees of pre-race arousal and each person interprets them differently. For some, symptoms of arousal signal excitement and readiness, while for others they cause increased anxiety that can negatively affect performance. Being too excited before a race is just as bad as being too subdued. Optimal competitive arousal varies from athlete to athlete, and your goal is to find a happy medium where you are psyched up to race, but not so amped that you're unable to eat on the morning of your race.

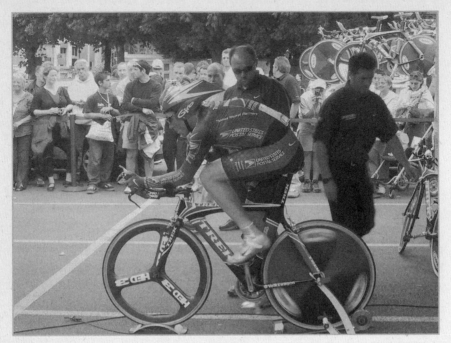

Lance Armstrong minutes before a Tour de France time trial. A good warmup includes both mental and physical preparation. *Photo © by Chris Carmichael*

Dealing with Over-Arousal Butterflies in the stomach, nausea, the inability to focus, cotton-mouth, and the constant need to urinate are all signs of increased arousal. In extreme cases, athletes are virtually incapacitated by their nerves. They're so emotionally overloaded that the decision to wear arm warmers or not can lead to a total meltdown. If this sounds familiar, you need to find a way to reduce your arousal on race day. Try one or more of the following techniques:

1. Centered breathing technique: This is a quick and effective way to calm down when you feel overexcited.
   a. Breathe in slowly to a count of three. As you breathe in, feel the air slowly filling your lungs.
   b. Slowly exhale to the count of three, letting the anxiety and stress flow out. You can also calmly and slowly say to yourself, *"Relax."*
   c. Repeat if necessary until you have reduced your level of arousal.

2. Relaxation: This is often time-dependent. Over-arousal can be compounded by being late or feeling rushed, so make a point to get to the race venue early. Instead of having to hurry to get ready to race, give yourself enough time to leisurely walk around the venue, lie in the grass, or take a nap.

3. Calming music: Music is extremely effective for helping athletes focus their attention, ignore distractions, and get into an optimal racing mind-set. Speed metal may not be the right music for you, though. Experiment with different music during your drives to race venues and during warmups.

Dealing with Under-Arousal When you're under-aroused before a race, your warmup is usually less effective, and you risk missing the start because you just aren't ready in time. The most extreme case of an under-aroused athlete I remember was when I was rolling to the start line and noticed a fellow competitor still asleep in his car. Apparently he woke up when we were halfway done with a 100-kilometer criterium. It is good to be calm and collected as you prepare to race, but your emotional activation also helps to trigger your physical activation. You don't want to "wake up" when the starting gun goes off, because your body will not react well to the sudden change from relaxation to race-intensity. If you normally feel sluggish and unfocused in the first five laps of a criterium, you may need to work on increasing your pre-race arousal. Try the following techniques:

1. Energizing breathing technique: This is a quick and effective way to psych yourself up when you don't feel like you have reached your optimal level of arousal.

   a. Inhale and exhale rapidly three times.

   b. As you inhale, feel the air filling your body, bringing with it a surge of energy.

   c. Exhale forcefully and quickly. You can also say, "*Go*" or "*Power*" to yourself each time you exhale.

   d. Repeat if necessary until you have increased your arousal level.

2. Watch others compete: Sometimes watching other people compete is enough to increase your excitement around racing. Let their high levels of arousal elevate your own.

3. Invigorating exercise: While I recommend that athletes warm up for events on a stationary trainer for improved consistency and effectiveness, under-aroused athletes may benefit from getting out on the road and going through some of the motions of bike racing. Take a few fast corners, sprint for a few street signs, and visualize the heat of competition. Some athletes also use activities like jumping jacks, push-ups, sit-ups, or pull-ups to increase their arousal.

4. Energetic music: Unlike the already over-aroused athlete, speed metal might be the music that works best for you. Try to find something with a constant and fast rhythm, and make the connection between the beat and your heart rate and cadence. Let the speed of the music infect you and psych you up.

One of the racers I knew and competed with was a part-time DJ at a dance club. He made his own mixes that matched the timing of his warmup. The beat of the music sped up and slowed down to correspond with the hard intervals and recovery time he built into his warmup routine. He used to say he heard the same pieces of music in his head during races, depending on the intensity of the effort he was putting out.

You can use an established routine for your pre-race activities to increase or decrease your arousal. If you have trouble with over-arousal, a routine can reduce the anxiety you feel around preparing to compete. Taking a step-by-step approach to registering, pinning on numbers, getting dressed, and warming up can help reduce your nervousness about forgetting to do something or making mistakes. If you are usually under-aroused, a routine can help you gradually increase your arousal level so you are ready to compete when the starting gun goes off. Your routine would integrate energizing activities or mental strategies into the standard steps of preparing for a race.

COMPETING AS THE 100% READY ATHLETE

Ride to win, not to avoid losing. This is your race, you're prepared for it, and you have the right and duty to do everything in your power to beat everyone else who shows up at the start line. That means you have to be smarter, more cunning, more careful, and more daring than everyone else. Arrive at the start line knowing you are prepared to beat everyone else standing with you.

Don't let the magnitude of the event, or the fact that this is your goal event, make you hesitant. There are some coaches who believe that athletes should approach all performances as if they are the same—as if there is no difference between a local training race and the National Championships. There is a difference, and you should use the magnitude of the event as a source of inspiration instead of anxiety. When you start a National Championship road race, you have the opportunity to finish the race in a Stars and Stripes jersey. You can't get that jersey next week, or next month, or whenever you happen to have a good day; it has to be today. The skills, legs, and lungs you use to compete in local races are the same tools you have to use to win a National Championship. You know how to use them and you know what to do to win bike races. Rely on the things you have already learned and practiced, use the tools you have as well as you can, and seize the opportunity to achieve your dreams.

Warm Up Like You Mean It

You have created a powerful aerobic giant through months of training and hard work, and your warmup must awaken that giant. A simple tap on the shoulder won't do it. You need to systematically activate your energy systems so you are entirely ready to compete when the starting gun goes off. While the first few miles of a road race may be relatively calm, you should be prepared to race hard from the start. Shorter events like criteriums and time trials begin hard and fast, and they generally stay that way.

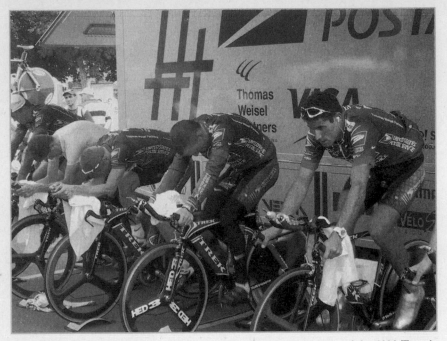

The U.S. Postal Service team warming up for the team-time-trial stage of the 2002 Tour de France. *Photo © by Chris Carmichael*

Initiate the Moves

Your experiences in training competitions have proven your ability to escape the peloton. You have also shown that you can be chased down and caught without being subsequently dropped. Allow those previous experiences to give you the confidence to launch off the front of the race. Initiating attacks has two purposes: (1) to form a solo or small group breakaway off the front and (2) to jettison excess baggage off the back. You are taking some control over the race when you are one of the people who force the pace, and you are making the race more difficult for everyone behind you. In the end, the smartest of the strongest racers in the field will win. You may be one of the strongest athletes in the peloton, but sitting in allows weaker racers to stay with you. The ability to make other racers work hard to keep up with you is part of your reward for months of hard work.

Be Attentive

You are not the only racer who has prepared specifically for this event, and there are other racers who want to win just as badly as you do. Don't let a lapse of concentration cost you your opportunity to win. Pay attention to what's going on around you and anticipate attacks and accelerations from your competitors. The quicker you react to their attacks, the less effort it takes to cover the move. You will expend less energy if you can accelerate with an attacker as opposed to having to bridge a gap or work your way back up to the front. Being attentive includes watching the road ahead and knowing the locations of significant climbs, feed zones, and prime sprints. Knowledge about your competitors is also helpful. In long road races and stage races, I recommend attaching course descriptions and certain racers' numbers onto your stem with tape. Having this information quickly available reduces the chance of being surprised to learn that you let a dangerous competitor get away in a break.

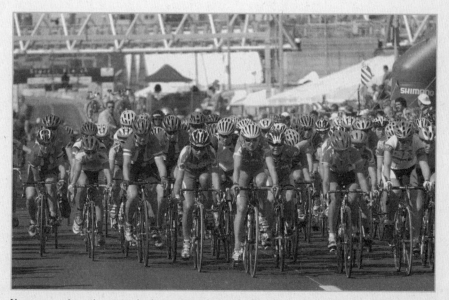

You are not the only racer who has prepared specifically for this event, and there are other racers who want to win just as much as you do. Pay attention and be ready to respond to attacks. *Photo © by Graham Watson*

Be Efficient

Win with your brain as well as with your legs and lungs. Watch the wind and stay in the draft when you can. Don't try to impress people with how much work you can do unless you will benefit from that work. Towing the breakaway to the line or pulling the entire field across a big gap benefits others more than it benefits you.

YOU CAN'T WIN IF YOU DON'T SPRINT

As I've said, "You can't win if you don't sprint" was a piece of advice given to me when I was nine years old following one of my first races in Miami. I had ridden well for the entire criterium and was in contention to win the race. When the sprint began, I got nervous because there were other racers close to me. I had a chance to win the race, but I lost it because I backed down at the critical moment. All the work I had done during the race to put myself in the position to win was in vain, because at the moment of truth I backed down and the winner didn't. That piece of advice changed the way I approached racing, and it helped me become a successful professional.

There are defining moments in every race. Looking back at the races you have competed in, can you find moments where your decision to stay put or follow wheels destroyed your chances of winning? Can you remember thinking, "Maybe I should go with that move," only to realize later that it was the winning move and a lost opportunity? It is better to lose a race as a result of trying to win it than to lose out of apathy. One way of controlling your own destiny in races is to cause the defining moment rather than waiting for someone else to do it for you.

Attack Hard, Make It Quick, and Be Gone

Attacking is a matter of commitment, so either attack with everything you have or don't go at all. To get away from the peloton, you have to accelerate so hard that others think twice before attempting to latch on to your wheel. Accelerate in the draft from somewhere in the first ten positions in the peloton. If you start from farther back, the riders at the front will have enough time to react to your acceleration before you pass them. Many riders attack to the opposite side of the road from the peloton to further discourage riders from following them. The effectiveness of this tactic depends on the conditions. On climbs, it is less important to attack to the side because of the decreased drafting effect. You want to accelerate straight ahead to create the bigger gap in less time. On flat ground, attacking to the side is more effective, but it may not be necessary to aim for the opposite edge of the road, especially on wide roads. For the first 30 seconds of your effort, keep your eyes on the road ahead of you. Looking back early is a sign to other riders that you don't really think you are going to be successful. Your immediate focus has to be on creating a gap, not on determining if there is anyone else with you. You undermine the effectiveness of your effort by focusing on too many things at once. First get away from the peloton, and then worry about how many riders are with you and your chances of staying away.

Attack When the Pace Is at Its Highest

This is a painful proposition, because your legs and lungs are already burning and I'm telling you to hit the throttle even harder. Remember, if you are hurting, so is the rider next to you. There are many instances where one more acceleration is all it will take to make the decisive selection. When riders are already struggling to keep up, they won't be able to accelerate and catch you. The reason riders hesitate to execute this tactic is the knowledge that they can't sustain such a high speed for long. But you don't have to. Once the selection is made, the pace of the breakaway and the main peloton usually falls to a fast but sustainable pace. You are attacking to cause the selection, and the riders you leave behind are there because you pushed them beyond their limits. They may be able to come after you once they recover, but by that time the gap will have grown, and bridging may again push them past their limits.

Attack Wisely

Where you choose to leave the peloton behind influences your chances of success. The general rule of thumb is to attack in a place where your effort will quickly result in a significant gap and maximize the effort required to bring you back.

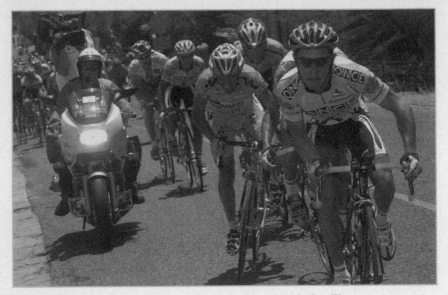

Launch your attack when the pace is at its highest. *Photo © by Graham Watson*

The Steepest Pitch Probably the single most effective place to attack is on the steepest pitch of a climb. You can put meters between yourself and your nearest competitor with every pedal stroke, and chasing you down takes an enormous effort from all involved. This is where you can take the greatest advantage of your power-to-weight ratio. Jan Ullrich was technically more powerful than Lance Armstrong in the 2001 Tour de France, but Lance had the advantage of being lighter. On flat ground, Lance would have had a hard time overpowering Ullrich; he may have gained some time, but he would have paid a huge cost for the effort. But in the mountains, Lance's lower weight gave him a higher power-to-weight ratio than the Deutsche Telekom team leader. To make the most of this advantage, Lance attacked on the steepest pitches of the climbs. He could accelerate uphill faster than Ullrich could, which meant he could establish significant gaps with relatively short accelerations. Once the gap was established, Lance settled into a fast but sustainable climbing rhythm. Eventually, Ullrich reached similar speeds on the climbs, but by the time he did, the damage was already done. He could limit his losses but not close the gap.

Countless champions have won their biggest races by attacking on climbs because the gaps that open are huge and it's possibly the most de-moralizing sight in cycling to see another rider sprint away from you when you are having trouble just keeping the pedals turning over. As ex-amples, look at Lance Armstrong on Beech Mountain in the 1996 Tour du Pont, the Manayunk Wall in the 1998 USPRO Championships (forced the winning selection), and Alpe d'Huez in the 2001 Tour de France. Repeated attacks on steep climbs also helped George Hincapie win the 2001 Ghent-Wevelgem and led to the final selection in the 2002 edition, where George and Freddy Rodriguez were beaten only by Mario Cipollini. And Will Frischkorn soloed to victory in the 2002 U23 National Championship road race by attacking on the steep pitch of the final climb to the finish. Push the pace on the climb, then put the final nail in people's coffins with a decisive attack at the hardest point.

Into a Corner Take advantage of the common deceleration before a corner to get away. Make a hard and quick acceleration off the front of the peloton in the straightaway shortly (50 to 75 meters) before a turn. The sharper and tighter the turn, the better this will work. The idea is to

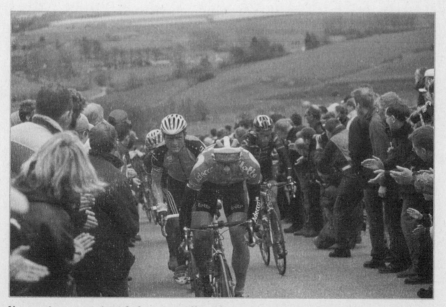

You get the greatest benefit from your effort when you attack on the steepest pitch of a climb.
Photo © by Graham Watson

get out in front so you can take the absolute fastest route through the turn. You're hoping the peloton is more cautious through the turn, giving you a critical few seconds to establish a gap. This is a risky move, because you are pushing your cornering skills and the laws of physics to their limits. If it works, you can win. If it doesn't, you may end up in the barriers. Again, this also works best when the corner's exit is uphill. You're carrying more momentum onto the climb, and the pitch makes it harder for anyone to accelerate up to you.

Out of Sight When the peloton can see you dangling just in front of them, they are motivated to come after you. If you're out of sight, you're out of mind and there's less motivation to chase you. On a long, straight road you have to be almost a minute ahead to be out of sight, so use a curvy or technically demanding section of road to establish your lead before emerging back onto open roads. Besides the factor of being out of sight, it is harder to organize an efficient chase through corners and urban areas. By the time the peloton gets organized, you're gone.

Repeat as Necessary More times than not, the peloton is going to chase you down. Realize that even though you were unsuccessful at forming a breakaway, the riders who chased you down had to dig into their energy reserves to catch you. You hurt their chances of winning the race each time you make them expend energy. That's energy they won't have the next time you launch off the front. This is where professional racers gain an advantage over amateurs. A professional uniform gives a racer a psychological advantage. Too often, amateur racers are too intimidated by the presence of professionals and they don't attack because they believe the professionals are too strong. In most American races, there are a handful of professionals competing against a majority of amateurs. The collective strength of the amateurs far outweighs the power of the pros. Attack them and make them earn their paychecks; don't give up just because of the jerseys they wear.

Bridging Gaps

Since you are not the only rider trying to win bike races, there will be times when you miss the break and have to bridge the gap from the peloton to the breakaway. The first thing to remember is not to panic; you can get across or help the peloton reel them back in. Since most amateur racers are racing for themselves, the notion of bringing a team to the front to bring back the breakaway is unrealistic. Your best move is to get across the gap and lend your support to the breakaway. Ideally, you are near the front when the attack happens and can accelerate with it. If you miss it by a few seconds, still go for it, but realize you have to attack even harder than the riders who initiated the attack, because you have some ground to make up. If you miss the attack completely, wait until the gap is small but established before you attempt to cross it. If the gap is too small, you may merely fill the hole between the fledgling breakaway and the peloton. Instead of bridging the gap and becoming part of the break-away, you will inadvertently pull the entire field up to the break. The breakaway needs to be far enough away that you can break contact with the riders behind you, cross an open space, and attach yourself to the front group.

If the gap has already grown to more than 20 seconds, your initial acceleration probably won't take you all the way across. Attack as if you are

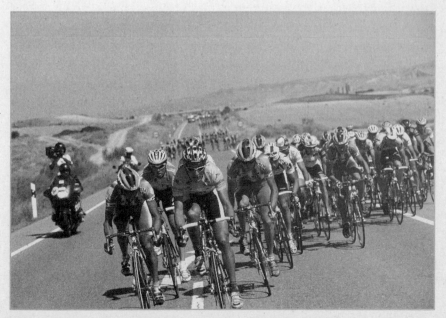

You have to act quickly to bridge gaps before they grow too big. *Photo © by Graham Watson*

initiating a move of your own and then quickly settle down into a pace higher than your normal time-trial pace. You will reach the breakaway only if you are going faster than they are, so for a period of one to two minutes you have to sustain a speed higher than that of the field and the breakaway. Be careful to maintain your effort as you approach the back of the breakaway. I've seen many riders start softpedaling too early, before they are actually in the breakaway's draft. They quickly lose momentum and have to accelerate again to close the final few meters. This small disruption of rhythm can be enough to prevent them from actually reaching the break.

Bridging gaps of more than one minute is very challenging. When you attack the peloton, you are committing to a sustained, all-out effort lasting several minutes. It is best to bring along some help to cross large gaps, essentially a second breakaway group chasing the first. You can share the work among several riders as you all pursue the leading group. Avoid the urge to attack your chasing partners as the distance to the breakaway decreases. If, as a group, you are gaining on the break, stick together until you get there. I know it's tempting to attack the chasers in hopes of reaching the breakaway without them, but you've come this far by working together. Attacking them may result in none of you reaching the break at all. It's better to reach the breakaway with a few more riders and have to tactically deal with a large breakaway group than to miss the opportunity to reach the break at all.

Whether you attempt to bridge a gap alone or with a small group, there is a chance that you will get stuck in no-man's-land. When you realize you are not gaining on the breakaway, you have to quickly assess the chances of successfully reaching them. If you are a strong climber and there is a significant hill coming up, keep going in the hopes of making up ground on the climb. But when you're stuck between the break and the peloton on flat ground or in the wind, your chances of regaining enough speed to start gaining on the break again are pretty slim. You may be better off going back to the peloton, regrouping and recovering, and trying again later. But make the decision quickly, because sitting 30 seconds in front of the peloton and 30 seconds behind the break for five minutes or more is a huge waste of energy.

FINISH IT OFF RIGHT

After making all the right moves in the beginning and middle of the race, make the last 20 kilometers of racing the best of your racing career. The final 25 minutes of racing is not the time to suddenly become hesitant or cautious. Riders start following wheels and racing conservatively as the finish approaches because they want to save energy for the finale. This is one of the reasons breakaways get caught within five kilometers of the finish. The peloton is chasing you and you're softpedaling! You've already shown that you have the power to attack and leave riders behind; why stop now? Go on the offensive and finish it. If the breakaway is playing games and not working well together, force the pace and make life difficult for the riders trying to sit on.

In criteriums you know what the finish looks like because you have crossed it dozens of times. But in road races, you may see the final five kilometers only once. I recommend inspecting the final five to ten kilometers of a road race-course so you know what to expect when the time comes. Knowing what the run-in to the finish looks like helps establish your tactical options. I learned the hard way. I attacked a breakaway with seven kilometers to go and established a pretty good gap. I thought I had the victory

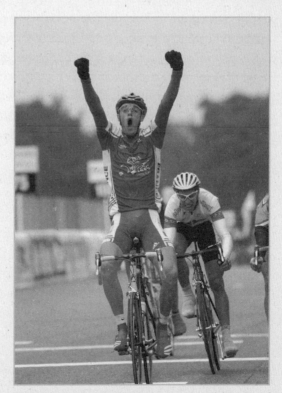

There's no feeling quite like crossing the finish line first.
Photo © by Graham Watson

in sight until I turned right, onto a steep 600-meter-long climb, with two kilometers to go. I had nothing left for the climb and watched in misery as the entire break caught and passed me as I reached the top. The winner knew about the climb and had waited until he reached it to launch the winning move.

Some racers can survive any race but never win anything. They're so focused on completing the race that they forget to try to win it. It may seem like a statement of the obvious, but if you've made it to the final 20 kilometers with the lead group, you're going to finish. Now you have to decide if you value finishing on the podium more than finishing in the field or off the back.

This is your goal event, the race you've spent the season preparing for. I tell my athletes I want them on the podium or off the back, but not somewhere in the middle. To win a bike race you have to risk losing it. Riders who refuse to take risks finish in the main field, but riders willing to put everything on the line become champions. By this time you know your strengths and weaknesses. Proactively set up a situation to best suit your strengths. If you are a strong sprinter, you want to keep the pace high to discourage attacks and keep the group together. If sprinting is not your strongest suit, a last-minute flyer may be your best chance for a win. Spoil the day for the sprinters and attack within the final two kilometers. All you need is a few seconds of hesitation from the group and you've won.

NUTRITIONAL CONSIDERATIONS FOR THE 100% READY ATHLETE

Nutrition plays a major role in your success as a 100% Ready Athlete. The nutrients you supply your body must provide fuel for performance as well as for recovery in order for you to compete optimally during your peak. Nutrient loading is part of your final preparation for your goal event. Loading nutrients is a process by which you optimize your body's ability to store and use energy. Carbohydrates are the most common nutrient that athletes load, but you can also benefit from loading fluids and fats.

Carbohydrate Loading

Glucose is the primary fuel for aerobic exercise, and endurance athletes benefit from eating a diet high in carbohydrates. You want to start your goal event with as much glucose as possible stored in your muscles as glycogen. One of the most effective methods of carbohydrate loading begins five to six days before your event. Decrease your carbohydrate intake to 50 percent of your caloric intake for two or three days. Three days before your goal event, go out on a long and moderately challenging ride to deplete your energy stores. Immediately following the long ride, increase your carbohydrate intake to 70 percent of your diet and maintain that level of intake until the morning of your event. This method of carbohydrate loading works extremely well in conjunction with the supercompensation ride I normally schedule for athletes three days before their goal events. That ride depletes the athletes' energy stores and leads to a short-lived state of fatigue. Since the overall training load is low, recovering from the ride is relatively easy and rapid. The body responds to the stress by overcompensating for the depletion of energy stores and storing more glycogen than normal. Be aware that your body stores three to five grams of water for every gram of carbohydrate it stores, so you may gain some weight as a result of carbohydrate loading. You should also try this technique several times during the season so you know how your body responds. Some people find they feel too bloated or sluggish to perform well, and even though they have more fuel, feeling sluggish and heavy can have a psychological effect that greatly diminishes performance. If carbohydrate loading works well for you, you should still try it several times throughout the season and experiment with different foods or drinks. Consuming a diet with 70 percent of the calories from carbohydrate can be very difficult without the use of supplements, and you should try different brands of carbohydrate drinks to determine which works best for you.

Fat Loading

Even the leanest athlete is storing enough fat calories to run a marathon, but accessing the energy is difficult. Considering the caloric density of fat (nine calories per gram) compared to glucose (four calories per gram), it would make more sense to burn fat for energy as opposed to carbohydrate. But you can process glucose from its storage form to usable energy much faster than you can process fat, making glucose a better fuel for exercise. Some people have advocated loading fat prior to extremely long endurance activities, especially events like RAAM (Race Across America), Iditasport, and 24-hour races. I don't believe that increasing your fat intake above your normal dietary level will lead to improved performance, but I do believe that you should be careful to maintain an adequate level of fat intake, even while carbohydrate loading. During carbohydrate loading, you are increasing the percentage of your total caloric intake coming from carbohydrate, but you should not completely drop fat or protein from your diet. The concept of fat loading may help some people avoid a drastic decrease in caloric intake from fats in the days prior to competition.

Protein Loading

Loading protein is not effective, because you don't have the ability to store it in the body as protein. Nearly all the tissues in your body are made from protein, and your body uses ingested protein for building new cells or converts it to glucose in the liver. Excess protein in the diet is simply excreted, and dealing with enormous amounts of excess protein can be hard on the kidneys. Ten to 15 percent of your total caloric intake should come from protein, even during carbohydrate loading.

Hydration: Water Loading

Adequate hydration is critical to performance, and it is an Achilles' heel for countless athletes. Many people are chronically dehydrated and don't realize that their performance can drastically improve just through fixing that one problem. But drinking a gallon of water the morning of your event won't do you much good, unless you normally drink that much. As with everything else, it takes some time for your body to adapt to consuming more fluids. Overcoming chronic dehydration can take days or weeks, because your body has adapted to function as well as possible on less water. Gradually increase your fluid intake, being careful to include some sports drinks as well as plain water. If you are not chronically dehydrated, you can still benefit from increasing your fluid consumption in the days prior to competition. Remember that each gram of carbohydrate stored in your muscles stores three to five grams of water with it, meaning that carbo-loading can lead to dehydration if you're not careful.

Excessive loading of fluids can lead to hyponatremia, or "water intoxication," a potentially fatal condition resulting from decreased concentrations of electrolytes in the body. Electrolytes, such as sodium, potassium, and calcium, help conduct the electrical charges essential for nervous-system function. Sodium is an electrolyte that is necessary for water balance, cellular metabolism, and muscular contractions. It draws water through permeable membranes and distributes fluid throughout the body. As you sweat, you are losing sodium and thus diminishing your body's ability to move water across these membranes. This will eventually lead to dehydration, even if you are drinking adequate amounts of water. Without sodium, the water you drink will not be distributed properly and you will feel bloated, nauseous, and unable to perform to the best of your ability. Other symptoms of hyponatremia include headaches, cramps, extreme fatigue, disorientation, and slurred speech. If these symptoms are allowed to progress, they can lead to seizures, coma, brain damage, and even death. You excrete large amounts of electrolytes through urine and sweat, and you must replenish them through eating and drinking. You can prevent hyponatremia by consuming sports drinks as well as water throughout all training sessions and competitions. During hot days in the Tour de France, riders may consume up to three bottles of fluid each hour they are racing, and approximately half the bottles they drink contain a sports drink. As with all aspects of nutrition and equipment, experiment with different brands of sports drinks during the season so you know what works best for you well before your goal event.

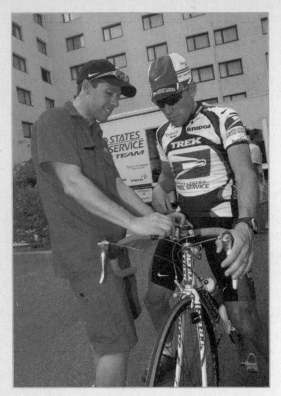

Lance Armstrong is famously meticulous when it comes to his bicycle. *Photo © by Graham Watson*

EQUIPMENT CHECK

You win bike races with your legs, lungs, brains, and determination; not because of the equipment you're riding. At the same time, broken and poorly maintained equipment can cost you the victories you worked so hard to achieve. You don't have to be a master mechanic to be a successful bike racer, but you should have enough working knowledge of bicycle mechanics that you can tell when there is something wrong with your machine. All of your equipment should be tested and proven well before your goal event. You should know what equipment you are going to use, right down to your water bottles, and that your equipment is in good working order.

1. Never make major repairs or changes the night before an event: This falls under the category of Golden Rules, never to be broken. If you inadvertently break something or make a mistake in adjusting your bike, you may not know about it until you are in competition. And many racing-eve changes aren't necessary anyway. I don't know how many times I've heard of someone crashing the morning after swapping out handlebars in the hotel room the night before. Cleaning and admiring are the only things you want to be doing to your bicycle the night before a race.

2. A clean bike is a fast bike: wash your bike before you race on it. A clean drive train is more efficient, and washing gives you the opportunity to inspect all parts of the bike. Check for frayed brake and derailleur cables, worn brake pads, and loose crank and chainring bolts. These are things you may not notice during normal training rides, and you wouldn't know about them until something breaks or falls off. Inspect your tires; cuts in the tread or sidewalls of your tires can lead to blowouts. Using separate sets of wheels for training and racing is one way of prolonging the life of expensive racing tires.

3. Lightweight equipment should be inspected and replaced frequently: all cycling equipment breaks eventually, so you should inspect your frame and components frequently for cracks and other signs of fatigue. Generally, the lighter the part, the more quickly it will fatigue. It is not that these parts are of poorer quality, it is just that there is a durability cost to manufacturing extremely lightweight components. If you choose to use extremely light parts, be prepared to replace them annually. The Lampre team learned this lesson in the 2002 Tour de France. They were using an old version of a lightweight aerobar on their time-trial bikes and three riders broke their bars during the team time trial. Since time trial bikes are rarely used, no one felt there was a need to replace the bars. Fortunately, no one crashed as a result of equipment failure, but the experience illustrates the need to regularly replace lightweight equipment.

Your Race Bag

Since you aren't busy repairing or modifying your bike the night before your race, you can spend some time preparing your race bag. Ideally, all you should have to do the morning of race day is throw things into the car and drive to the venue. You will invariably forget something when you try to pack your bag on the morning of the race.

Pack clothing for all types of weather, because conditions change rapidly and unpredictably. One hot July day in Wisconsin, it looked like we would start a road race in blazing sun. Less than 30 minutes before the start, strong thunderstorms on the leading edge of a cold front pushed over us. Those of us who had rain and cool-weather gear in our race bags simply put on a few layers of clothes and reported to the start line. Many riders weren't prepared for the weather change; nearly one third of the field either didn't start or failed to finish just due to the weather. Besides normal things like your helmet, uniform, shoes, and first-aid kit, your race bag should always include:

1. *Clothing*
   a. Arm warmers, leg warmers
   b. Long- and short-fingered gloves
   c. Rain/wind gear. Always pack a rain cape as well as a wind-resistant vest or jacket. These garments are good outer shells to layer on top of your uniform in inclement weather. They are also small enough to be stuffed into your jersey pocket if the weather clears up.
   d. Shoe covers, preferably medium-weight and water-resistant. You're going to want these if you have to race in the rain, so you don't want the aerodynamic shoe covers that offer no insulation. Nor do you need the super-warm thermal booties you use to ride through the snow.
   e. Base layers. The clothing layer closest to your skin is very important. Bring a layer designed for racing in hot weather, and another one designed for cold weather. Your cold-weather base layer should be long-sleeved, and you may want to purchase one with a wind-resistant fabric in the front. See Chapter 6 for more information on clothing layers.
   f. Sunglasses and lenses. I recommend at least three options for eyewear: a clear lens, an orange (persimmon) or yellow lens, and a dark lens. These three lens options cover a wide range of light conditions. Dr. Rick Kattouf, an optometrist and CTS member, recommends that cyclists and multi-sport athletes always wear some form of eyewear while exercising outdoors. As a member of the U.S. National Duathlon Team, Dr. Kattouf sees eyewear as a necessary piece of sporting equipment, just like shoes and a helmet. He says, "Modern eyewear offers protection from UVA and UVB rays, as well as foreign objects. In some cases, colored lenses can improve an athlete's ability to

see contrast and distinguish objects in either bright light or low-light conditions."

2. *Extra/Spare Parts*

g. Tires and tubes. If you are riding clincher tires, always bring at least one extra tire and two extra tubes. If you are racing on tubular tires, bring a spare set of wheels, preferably with clincher tires on them. If you flat a tubular tire while warming up for your race, you won't be able to remount a new tubular tire in time to safely race on it.

h. Brake cables, derailleur cables, and brake pads. Broken cables and missing brake pads are extremely rare problems, but any one of them will prevent you from starting a race. These parts take up very little room in your race bag, and in the rare instance you need them, you will be very thankful to have them with you.

i. Spokes. Carrying your own spokes and spoke nipples is especially important if you compete with specialty wheels. Depending on where you are racing, you may have trouble finding a bike shop with spokes to fit your wheels. If fixing your wheels requires special tools, bring those with you also.

j. Cleats. Always have an extra set of cleats with you. The cleats on your shoes wear out, so eventually you'll need to install a new pair anyway. In the meantime, you'll have the extras with you in case your current ones break.

k. Bar Plugs. According to USA Cycling rules, you must have plugs in the ends of your handlebars in order to compete. They are easy to lose, and it is just as easy to pack an extra pair in your bag.

THE FEED ZONE

Feed zones aren't much of a consideration for many racers because there is no feeding in criteriums or time trials, nor in road races under 50 kilometers. However, for those of you competing in longer road races and mountain bike races, here's some useful feed-zone etiquette:

1. Start the race with enough food to get through the entire event if you have to. You may not get your feed, and a few energy bars aren't really that heavy. It may be difficult to carry enough water for an entire race because bottles are bulky and heavy, so make fluid replacement your first priority in the feed zone.

2. Find out about neutral support. Neutral support can consist of mechanical support and spare wheels, and it can also include water bottles in the feed zone. Many times this means bottled water with a screw-cap. They probably won't fit in your bottle cages; just stuff a few in your jersey and deal with them later.

3. If you are going to have someone in the feed zone, pack a bag with real food as well as energy bars or gels. Experiment with different types of sandwiches and fruit during training rides so you know what works best for you. Snacks like fig bars are also good because they are good sources of complex carbohydrates.

4. If you are feeding, get in line. If you are not, get to the left side of the road. The feed zone can be chaotic, and getting out of the way reduces your probability of being involved in a crash.

5. If you miss your feed, your feeder should never throw a bottle after you.

6. Find your feeder, don't make him find you. Try to establish where you will meet (beginning, end, or middle of the zone). Feeders should wear recognizable clothing. Sometimes team jerseys are not the best choice because several jerseys may look very similar.

7. Tip for feeders: Keep the bottle or bag close to you and keep your eyes open. Opportunistic riders will steal your rider's bag if you make it easy. Extend the food out only when your rider approaches.

8. Be nice to your feeder. Standing in the feed zone all day and trying to get bottles to you is a pain in the butt and pretty boring. If you miss your feed or get the wrong bottle, live with it and be grateful someone was there to even try to get something to you.

9. Do what you have to do.
   a. Snagging a water bottle is risky but not against the rules. If you miss your feeder, snag someone's bottle before leaving the

feed zone. Be quick. If the feeder sees you reaching for the bottle, he or she will pull it back. Reach out at the last second and snatch it.

b. Trade food for water. If you are carrying some extra food, you can try to trade it for water. You don't know if someone else has the opposite problem you do: enough water but not enough food.

Talking about feed zones in races inevitably leads us to waste management. The pros set a bad example by tossing bottles and wrappers along the roadside, and there is really no good excuse for them or you to continue doing so. When you are done with your PowerBar,® put the wrapper back in your jersey and throw it out after the race. If you're worried about a leftover-goopy-PowerGel mess in your jersey pocket, tuck the wrapper into the leg elastic of your shorts; I promise it won't affect your performance. It may be necessary to jettison water bottles during a race, and you should do so in places where they can be recovered. You need to make sure to drop or toss your bottle off to the side of the road, but there's no need to hurl it into the next county. Get rid of your bottle(s) within sight of the feed zone so race volunteers can leave the area as clean as they found it. Litter is one of the objections that race promoters encounter from residents and city officials when they try to organize events. Please act responsibly so the promoters can continue to provide opportunities to compete.

COMPETITIVE ENVY

A rider's reputation sometimes lends her more power than she actually possesses. There may be a cyclist who is regarded as the top sprinter in your region, or the top climber, or simply the fastest racer overall. That distinction should never preclude you from challenging him or her. Back in the 1980s when the 7-Eleven team competed in Pro-Am™ races in the States, the amateurs made it easy for us to win because they backed down instead of challenging us for wheels. As I made the transition to coaching, I tried to instill my athletes with the idea that they have the right to fight anyone for any wheel. Don't give way to another racer simply because of his reputation or the jersey on his back. If he has the skills and speed to outride you, he will do so whether you challenge him or not, so you might as well challenge him. Your racing experience, your talent, and your hard work have given you the right to hold your ground. Don't grant privileges to other riders they wouldn't extend to you.

You may not have the amenities that other racers on large teams have. Maybe there's no one waiting in the feed zone for you, and no one waiting for you after the race with food and a change of clothes. You don't have a soigneur to rub down your legs before and after events, to fill your water bottles, or help you with your gear. Instead of envying the pros for the amenities they have, revel in your self-sufficiency. Be proud that you can compete with and beat riders who receive more assistance than you do. The committed amateur bike racer is the heart and soul of bike racing. The skills and fortitude you learn as a solitary racer affect your outlook on life for a long time.

HOW LONG CAN YOU REMAIN 100% READY?

When everything comes together and you have the ability to race as a 100% Ready Athlete, you can compete at a level you've never experienced before. It's a feeling you never want to relinquish, but all good things must eventually come to an end. The length of time complete readiness can be maintained varies from athlete to athlete, and it is important to make the most of your time on top and recognize the signs of your decline.

All athletes have a window of time when they can compete at an optimal level. During this period, you can maintain your focus on all aspects of performance, including fitness, coordination, recovery, competitive drive, hydration, and nutrition. Eventually, the strain of competition wears you down and things begin to slip. I have found that almost all athletes can be 100% Ready for about four weeks, and that their focus on nutrition and recovery is the first thing to start declining. Remaining attentive to all aspects of cycling means carefully considering how every minute of your day relates to your competitive form. This level of intensity is difficult to maintain, and your activities off the bike are often the first places you will lose focus. Unfortunately, lapses in recovery and nutrition seriously affect your ability to continue performing at optimal levels, and soon your racing performance starts to suffer. While this is frustrating for athletes to experience, it is a perfectly natural and necessary process. The important thing is to make the most of your form when you have it and plan your goal events carefully.

More experienced athletes can extend the duration of their 100% Readiness to about seven or eight weeks. This ability is developed by years of competition and training and is the result of physical and psychological adaptations. Fitness is cumulative, and over a period of years you can gradually raise your level of peak conditioning as well as your physical ability to cope with the strain of racing. Your body becomes increasingly efficient in using fuel and replenishing depleted energy sources. Your muscles and connective tissues also increase in strength and in resistance to breakdown, which means they can withstand longer periods of high-intensity racing. Handling the psychological strain of racing is a matter of learning the mental strategies that work best for you. In your first few years of racing, it is difficult to know exactly what to expect from weeks of continued high-intensity racing. Once you have experienced the ups and downs of competition a few times, you are better prepared to handle the strain in following seasons.

Dave Zabriskie and Lance Armstrong are both extremely talented athletes, but Lance has several more years of experience than Dave does. In 2002, Lance started the season as a three-time defending Tour de France Champion and Dave had never completed a single three-week Grand Tour. Having worked with both athletes for several years, I knew Lance had the ability to be 100% Ready for around seven weeks, while Dave's readiness would last only three to four weeks. Dave's situation was similar to Lance's in the early 1990s. Back then, Lance could maintain top performance for only about four weeks before his motivation and attention to detail started to slip. Each time we prepared for a peak, Lance and I worked on a different aspect of top performance, focusing particularly on nutrition during one peak and working on competitive drive during the next. Not only did his physical training lead to new heights of performance with each successive peak, the educational processes we employed helped him hold on to his 100% Readiness longer each time. I believe an athlete needs to be able to maintain optimal form for at least six weeks to be a Grand Tour contender, and Lance reached that stage of development in 1998. That year he finished fourth in the Tour of Spain, and the next year he won his first Tour de France.

The level and duration of Dave Zabriskie's peaks have been increasing gradually over the past four years, and in 2002 he was able to maintain top performance long enough to complete his first Grand Tour, the Tour of Spain. Finishing your first Grand Tour is a rite of passage for professional cyclists. It is the most difficult challenge you have ever faced, and completing one changes you physically and mentally. The 2002 Tour of Spain was an important stepping-stone for Dave, because he had to learn to cope with the enormous physical and mental pressures involved in such an event. As we prepare for subsequent peaks, he has the experiences and knowledge he gained during that event to build upon. Riders do not begin their careers with the ability to complete or win Grand Tours; the necessary skills must be gained through years of cumulative growth and development.

Training builds upon itself, both in your ability to handle load from week to week and in the heights of performance you can reach from year to year. Working closely with a coach helps you get the most out of your training to develop the skills to reach and maintain top performance during a peak.

CTS coach James Herrera worked with CTS Member John C. for several months before the first organized peaking process of John's cycling career. John was preparing for a multi-day cycling tour, and he and James spent a lot of time during the peaking process working on John's recovery habits. In the evenings during the tour, John recalled the things he and his coach had discussed and as a result he rode as well on the last day of the tour as on the first. John decided he wanted to ride a similar tour later in the same season, so James developed a plan for John to peak a second time a few months later. Since they had already worked on John's recovery habits, John and James decided to focus on hydration and nutrition during his next peaking process. Following his second multi-day tour, John told us in a CTS Member Report that his friends were amazed at how fresh and strong he rode during the very hilly fourth and final day of the tour. John had successfully used the skills he had developed through two peaking processes to have the best experience of his cycling career.

The process of developing into a 100% Ready Athlete is not an end unto itself. Rather, it is a step in the ongoing process of developing into a more complete athlete. Each time you follow an organized training plan and achieve the goals you have set for yourself, you learn valuable lessons that you will benefit from the next time you prepare for a peak.

11

After the Peak

AFTER SPENDING MONTHS PREPARING, focusing, and sacrificing for your goal event, it's perfectly natural to be emotionally connected to the race. That emotional connection helped you compete at your best, and now that the event is over, you have to deal with the consequences of winning or losing.

Some athletes, whether they win or lose, immediately put the event behind them and move on to the next goal. That's not the way you deal with other emotional events in your life, so why would it be the right way to deal with this one? When you graduated, landed a great job, or got married, you took time to celebrate and recognize the achievement. And when you broke up with your first serious girlfriend or boyfriend, lost someone close to you, or got laid off from that great job, you took time to be angry or mournful. When you work hard to achieve something or make something work, there is an emotional attachment to succeeding or failing.

Passionate athletes have a higher capacity for success, and the way you deal with your race results can affect your overall passion for the sport. Early in Lance Armstrong's career, his goals were somewhat vague. He wanted to be a top professional racer, but he didn't feel passionately about any particular event. He had goals around preparing for the Classics, the Tour de France, the World Cup, and the World Championships. He wanted to win as many races as he could, but win or lose, as soon as one race was over, he just looked ahead to the next one. He taught himself not to take the good or bad races personally, and that robbed him of the passion it takes to win races. It led to reduced commitment around his next goal and less overall passion for the sport.

Stopping long enough to recognize success and failure was one of the many changes that cancer caused in Lance's approaches to racing. Instead of suppressing the disappointment of losing a race, Lance started expressing it and dealing with it. He allowed himself to get sad and pissed-off about defeats, and he started celebrating his victories. He started to let the emotional connections to racing grow; he really started enjoying the process and results of training and racing. I believe that an athlete's passion for the sport is nurtured by his or her emotional interaction with goals, successes, and failures. Lance's passion for cycling motivates him to put in the hours of training necessary to prepare him for success in the Tour de France.

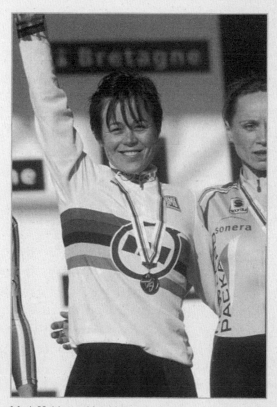

Mari Holden achieved her dream after more than six years of hard work. *Photo © by Graham Watson*

COPING WITH SUCCESS

Celebrate your achievement and take credit for the things you accomplished through hard work and determination. Something odd happens to some athletes when they win; all of a sudden the event that was so important to them diminishes in meaning. Groucho Marx was famous for saying he wouldn't want to join any club that would have him as a member, and some athletes seem to share that sentiment. Any race they could win really couldn't have been very important or difficult. Your success should not be based on the grandeur of the race, but on the fact that you set out to accomplish a goal, worked hard to prepare yourself, and then went out and did it.

Allow your achievement to boost your confidence and motivate you to pursue new goals. The first time you truly realize one of your goals, the experience can change the way you approach cycling. This sport sometimes seems like it is predicated on luck above all else; that success is more of a crapshoot than something you can control. Success in racing confirms that you *really do* know what you're doing, and this confirmation is very important for improving self-confidence. When you look at future racing goals and say, "Yeah, I can do that. I know how to do that," you have the confidence to succeed repeatedly. If you believe that your success was due to a lucky rabbit's foot attached to your race bag, a special undershirt, or a good-luck kiss from your spouse, then you have abdicated responsibility for your actions and decisions in competition. You can't gain confidence from a goal when you give away the responsibility and credit for accomplishing it. Achieving your goals is similar to getting a power-boost in a computer game; you win one round and you get a power-boost that lets you start the next round with added strength and abilities.

Now that I have encouraged you to pump up your ego, let me also encourage you to keep your success in perspective. Success in racing means you trained and competed well, and that on that day you were the best competitor. It doesn't mean:

1. You're going to win everything, or even your next race.
2. Everyone around you expects you to win everything.

3. You can stop working as hard as you have been.
4. You're better than the rest of the field.

For some athletes, accomplishment leads to anxiety about their abilities to ever succeed again. This is natural, especially after performing better than ever before. The questions you may ask include: "Was that the best performance I will ever have?" "Will I ever be able to ride that well again?" and "Will I ever get to experience this feeling again?" There's absolutely no way you can definitively answer those questions, so you might as well answer them positively. No, that wasn't your best performance. It was just your best performance so far. Yes, you will be able to ride that well again. Chances are, you're going to ride even better in the future. And finally . . . yes, you will get to experience again the wonderful feeling of accomplishing what you set out to do. Write down as much as you can remember about your day and carry the benefits of your success forward to your next goal.

Coping with Not Meeting Your Goal

Highly motivated people set challenging goals because they find value in overcoming the challenge. Setting a lofty goal means increasing the risk that you won't quite reach it, but also increasing the value and sense of achievement you get when you do reach it. When you are in the situation of not having met your goal, and you will eventually find yourself in that situation, allow yourself to be disappointed, deal with it, and then use the experience to enhance your pursuit of your next goal.

In the same manner in which athletes diminish the value of races after they win, people tend to quickly dismiss poor performances as well. I agree that you shouldn't spend too much time dwelling on missed opportunities and what might have been, but you spent a lot of time and energy preparing for this event and it is good to recognize your disappointment with not meeting your goals. When you train yourself not to care about great and poor performances, your race results gravitate toward the middle: nothing great, nothing terrible, and everything in the middle of the field. A dispassionate attitude about results leads to decreased attention to training and competition. If achievement doesn't make you feel great, and if not meeting your goals doesn't bother you, how invested

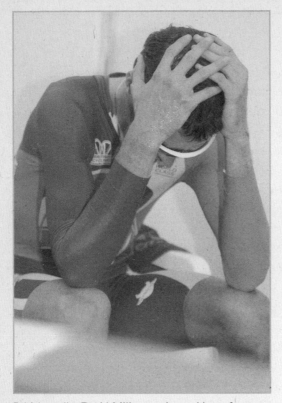

British cyclist David Millar reacting to his performance after being narrowly beaten in the Time Trial World Championship. *Photo © by Graham Watson*

and personally committed are you to what you're doing? It's tempting to be stoic about race results because it is easier than riding the emotional roller-coaster of a cycling season, but I believe that an emotional attachment to training and competition improves your performance. I've seen hundreds of athletes with the numeric strength and power to be successful professional cyclists, and the handful that have been the most successful are the ones who deeply care about their performances during every training session and competition.

Be careful not to equate not meeting your goal with failure. Although I believe that it is best to make specific goals, it's also a dangerous practice, because the more specific your goal, the smaller the chance that you can achieve it. Winning a race on August 19 is a far more specific goal than racing competitively in August, but the latter is easier to achieve. But you are not a failure just because you didn't win on August 19. Look at the bigger picture. You may not have won the race, but did you perform better than ever before? Did you do everything in your power to win the race? Peaking for your goal event taught you important lessons for growing as an athlete, and as long as you are continuing the process of growth, you can't fail. Treasure your best performances and accept your worst, because they are all part of your development.

While it is important to deal with being disappointed about not meeting your goal, you also have to put it behind you and proceed with training and racing. It is alright to be disappointed in your decisions, your performance, and your result; but it's a bike race, not the end of the world. And look what good came of the endeavor: you are more fit than ever before, you have another several months of cumulative training under your belt, and you have the experience of completing at least one peaking process. Now you can move on and further refine the process for subsequent goals. Take note of the things you can improve in your next race, or in the process of reaching your next peak. Talk with a coach or someone close to you and share your ideas of what went well and what needs to be improved. Then accept the poor result as a fact of the past and move on.

LEARNING FROM ONE RACE TO THE NEXT

The learning curve in cycling is one of the major reasons why the average age of Tour de France champions is 29 years. Most racers have at least a decade of racing experience before even being considered a contender for a race as complicated as the Tour de France. No two races are the same, and there are lessons you can take from every competition. What has made Erik Zabel, Robbie McEwen, and Mario Cippolini the dominant sprinters of their generation? There are other riders who can match their speed and power, but few who can match their knowledge of how to win sprint finishes. Their superlative ability is based on thousands of race finishes and the knowledge they gained from each one.

Winning bike races is a matter of being fit and knowing how and when to apply your strength. This is one of the reasons I recommend waiting to upgrade your racing category until you win at least three races in your current category. As you move up from Category 5 to Category 1, contending for victory becomes more challenging. It is important to learn how to win early in your racing career, because once you develop the skills, winning at any level is just a matter of gaining more power and applying your skills at higher speeds.

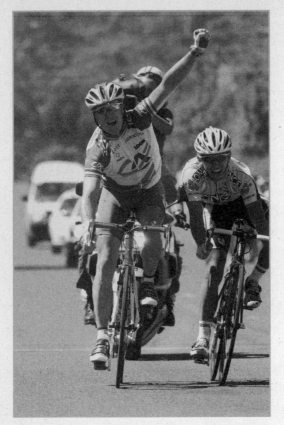

Stuart O'Grady winning the 2003 Australian National Road Race Championships. He has honed his ability to win races through years of experience.
Photo © by Graham Watson

The best way to learn from your races is to write down as much as you can remember about the decisions that improved or hindered your chances of victory. This includes pre-race activities like your pre-race meal, warmup routine, and clothing and equipment selections. Replay the race in your head and consider the consequences of your decisions. You shouldn't necessarily assign value judgments to your decisions; just write down the facts of what happened. Afterward, read through the story and pinpoint the places where your decisions improved or hindered your chances of winning. Read the following account from a road race and figure out where you made mistakes:

You went with an early breakaway, and although you were caught, half the field was dropped in the process. You missed your feed because you couldn't find your girlfriend in the feed zone, and even though you managed to get a neutral water bottle, you ran out of food with 70 kilometers to go. You attacked the field 20 kilometers from the finish, but five kilometers from the start of a large climb. By the top of the climb, your 30-second advantage had turned into a 40-second deficit with ten kilometers to go. You gathered a group of chasers on the descent and you all worked together to rejoin the lead group two kilometers from the finish. One rider from your chase group attacked straight past the leaders as you caught them. Everyone looked at one another, waiting for someone to ignite the chase, and that lone rider crossed the finish line by himself. As you entered the final turn and into the sprint for second place, you decided to dive to the inside of the turn because you saw an opportunity to move up. You didn't know about the sunken manhole cover in the middle of that turn, though, and you barely managed to keep the bike upright as you slammed both wheels through it. Even though you regained control of your bike, the riders who took the outside line through the turn had a lot more momentum going into the sprint. You dug deep for the power to sprint, but your legs just couldn't respond. Two hundred meters later, you were the last finisher from the lead group.

It's a good result, a top-ten finish in the State Championship road race, but what could you have done differently to improve your chances of winning?

The good things you did:

1. You were in the early breakaway.
2. You quickly grabbed a neutral water bottle when you realized you had missed your feed.
3. You took the race into your own hands by attacking 20 kilometers from the finish.
4. You organized a chase group to rejoin the leaders instead of racing for fifth place.
5. You looked for and took advantage of what looked like an opportunity to win the sprint for second place by diving to the inside of the final turn.

Based on the list of good things you did, I would consider this a successful race, regardless of the final result. You raced aggressively and were a factor in the race from beginning to end.

Things that hindered your chances of winning:

1. You couldn't find your girlfriend in the feed zone.
2. You started the race without enough food to make it to the finish, so you ran low on fuel at the end of the race.

3. You attacked the field at an inopportune point of the race.
4. You didn't gather enough information about the race to know about the five-kilometer climb 15 kilometers from the finish.
5. You chose not to chase the lone rider who attacked with two kilometers to go.
6. You didn't pre-ride the run-in to the finish, so you didn't know about the manhole cover.

You can deal with most of the things that hindered your chances of winning by planning ahead before your next race. Have your feeder wear distinctive clothing, and have her stand in a predetermined section of the feed zone. Start the race with enough food to get to the finish; it doesn't weigh very much. Learn as much as you can about the course, including the positions of all the major climbs and the characteristics of the run in to the finish. Two of your tactical decisions didn't work out as well as you had hoped, and that's important to remember for future races. Neither your attack five kilometers before the last major climb, nor your choice to let the lone attacker go with two kilometers left in the race, was necessarily wrong. In different circumstances, either one of those decisions may have helped you win. As you accumulate more racing experience, you will learn what tactics, and what circumstances, combine for great results. But you'll only gain that knowledge by carefully examining each performance.

SPORTS PSYCHOLOGY WORKSHEETS

The CTS coaches and I use the following worksheets with some CTS members to help them identify their strengths and weaknesses in competition. The first worksheet is especially useful for reminding athletes of their goals for specific races, and of the methods they plan on using to achieve those goals. The Post-Competition Reflection Worksheet is a good way to record race results as well as the factors that led to that result. It also helps to ask the same questions after each event so you can more easily compare the answers. After you have been racing for a while, you can look back at Post-Race Reflections from your first races and see how much you have developed.

Determining Your Optimal Race Environment

example

Consider your best and worst performances and answer the following questions. Review your answers with your coach to help determine how you can best prepare for competition.

I. Think of your all-time BEST cycling performance or performances.

1. How did you feel just before the race started?

| VERY PHYSICALLY CHARGED | 1 | 2 | 3 | (4) | 5 | VERY PHYSICALLY RELAXED |

| VERY MENTALLY CHARGED | 1 | 2 | (3) | 4 | 5 | VERY MENTALLY RELAXED |

| NOT VERY WORRIED | 1 | (2) | 3 | 4 | 5 | VERY WORRIED/ ANXIOUS |

2. What were you saying to psyche yourself up before the start of the race?
   I can't wait, what a fantastic day, this course is awesome.

3. Were you focusing on your team, yourself, or your competitors prior to the race?
   Talking to teammates

4. What things in your environment (music, people, etc.) helped psyche you up?
   My teammates, lots of people/spectators

example

5. What kind of warmup did you do?

20-min spin with teammates with one or two jumps, stretched

II. Think of your all-time WORST cycling performance or performances.

1. How did you feel just before the race started?

VERY PHYSICALLY CHARGED	1	②	3	4	5	VERY PHYSICALLY RELAXED

VERY MENTALLY CHARGED	1	2	3	④	5	VERY MENTALLY RELAXED

NOT VERY WORRIED	1	2	3	④	5	VERY WORRIED/ ANXIOUS

2. What were you saying to psyche yourself up before the start of the race?

Crap—look who's here, those hills are going to kill me, I'm not ready.

3. Were you focusing on your team, yourself, or your competitors prior to the race?

Thinking of competitors

4. What things in your environment (music, people, etc.) helped psyche you up?

Not a lot of teammates were there, so I was distracted by other teams.

5. What kind of warmup did you do?

20-min spin alone with one or two jumps, stretched

III. Now compare your responses to these two scenarios and indicate how you would like to feel prior to competition.

_____

_____

_____

_____

_____

_____

_____

_____

_____

_____

PRE-PLANNING FOR COMPETITION example

Race name, location, time, and date: *Harvard 100k, Harvard, MA on 06/15 12:30 P.M.*

Am I going to pre-register? N/Y—send application by _____/

Transportation to the race? *I am driving, taking Jane and Kim. Jane has directions.*

Before leaving for the race:
- *Review race-bag checklist to make sure I have all equipment—pack night before.*
- *Call Jane and Kim at 6:30 A.M. to make sure they are up.*
- *Bike/cooler/race bag/spare wheels/tool kit in car.*

Once I arrive at the race site:
- *Check in and get race number.*
- *Get bike ready/quick check of brakes, etc.*

My warmup routine—what do I need to do to get properly prepared, and how much time do I need?
- *Need one hour after check-in.*
- *Check bike over, change clothes.*
- *5 to 20 minute spin with two good jumps (ride with teammates who are ready).*
- *Check in with teammates to see how everyone is feeling—talk about QOM and possible primes—who is up for them?*
- *Drink at least one bottle of water.*
- *Spend five minutes alone stretching/relaxing after riding but at least 20 minutes before start.*
- *Get to start line at least five minutes early.*

example

My competition goals (performance and outcome) are:

- *Want to get in top three for QOM (last year 4th—one out of $!!).*
- *Consistent with pack but no "coasting" mid-race.*

My race plan (how do you plan to accomplish your goals) is:

- *Have two intensity checkpoints in race—one right after the finish and one right before each lap before the "BIG" hill.*
- *For QOM—check positioning in half-mile before the "BIG" hill.*

What are possible distractions, and what will I do about them (e.g., arriving late, flatting in the race)?

- *Brought spares for wheel pit.*
- *Jane and Kim are going to help me with QOM positioning.*
- *Calling Jane and Kim to ensure we leave on time.*

POST-RACE REFLECTIONS *example*

Consider your race as objectively as possible. Use this sheet to help further understand the things that help you perform well and the things that get in your way.

Race name: *Superweek Madison State Building Crit in Madison, WI*
Weather: *Chilly, low 50s, nasty wind*
Length of Race: *25 miles (1.2-mile course)*
Field Size: *55 riders*   Place: *15th in field sprint and one prime*

How did you perform during the race? Were you able to accomplish your race goals?
Kept up my intensity and played it very well with the headwind on the back side of the course.
Took one prime, but had a poor position for the field sprint.

What things positively impacted your ability to perform?
Having Jon lead me out for the prime worked really well!
Cornering practice earlier in the season seems to be paying off, too.

What things negatively impacted your performance—and what could you do to prevent or deal with these things in the future?
- *Not properly prepared for cold—had trouble with hands and toes toward end of the race—need to keep some warm riding gear in race bag even midsummer.*

What did you learn from this performance? Physically, technically, tactically, mentally?
- *Still need more cornering work, especially setting up for a field sprint one or two corners before the finish line in a tight crit like this.*
- *Need to remember to work on positive self-talk when something goes wrong.*

example

What would you do the same to prepare for your next competition?

• *I prepared for this race really well—I got there in plenty of time, had a good warmup, and followed my pre-race plan.*

What would you do differently in preparing for your next competition?

• *Be more prepared for weird weather changes, but other than that my pre-race warmup went really well this time.*

PRE-PLANNING FOR COMPETITION worksheet

Race name, location, time, and date: _____

Am I going to pre-register? N/Y—send application by _____

Transportation to the race? _____

Before leaving for the race:
- *Review race-bag checklist to make sure I have all equipment* _____
- _____
- _____

Once I arrive at the race site:
- *Check in and get race number* _____
- _____
- _____

My warmup routine—what do I need to do to get properly prepared, and how much time do I need? _____
_____
_____

My competition goals (performance and outcome) are: _____
_____
_____

My race plan (how do you plan to accomplish your goals) is: _____
_____
_____

What are possible distractions, and what will I do about them? (e.g., arriving late, flatting in the race) _____
_____
_____

POST-RACE REFLECTIONS worksheet

Consider your race as objectively as possible. Use this sheet to help further understand the things that help you perform well and the things that get in your way.

Race name: _____

Weather: _____

Length of Race: _____

Field Size: _____ Place: _____

How did you perform during the race? Were you able to accomplish your race goals?

_____

_____

_____

_____

What things positively impacted your ability to perform?

_____

_____

_____

_____

What things negatively impacted your performance—and what could you do to prevent or deal with these things in the future?

_____

_____

_____

_____

worksheet

What did you learn from this performance? Physically, technically, tactically, mentally?

_____

_____

_____

_____

What would you do the same to prepare for your next competition?

_____

_____

_____

_____

What would you do differently in preparing for your next competition?

_____

_____

_____

_____

Glossary of Abbreviations

CR: ClimbingRepeats; These are similar to SS, except they are performed while climbing at slightly lower cadences. CR efforts improve power at climbing lactate threshold. As a result, the CR heart rate range is closer to the individual's time trial heart rate.

DI: DescendingIntervals; a series of progressively shorter intervals and equally short recovery times. Designed to increase your anaerobic power, lactate tolerance, and repeatability during maximum efforts. pp. 96–97

EM: EnduranceMiles; one of the fundamental workouts for endurance cyclists. Most of your interval workouts will occur within EM rides. pp. 97–98

FP: FastPedal; a workout designed to improve pedaling mechanics and efficiency. pp. 98–99

FG: FixedGear; a ride performed on a fixed-gear bicycle. These bicycles don't allow you to coast. As long as the wheels are moving, you have to pedal. pp. 99–100

FM: FoundationMiles; one of the fundamental workouts for endurance cyclists. These rides are at a slightly lower intensity and pace than EnduranceMiles. Many of your rides in the Foundation Period will be at FM intensity. pp. 100–101

HSS: HighSpeedSprints; a sprint workout during which each sprint begins at high speed to simulate racing finishes and increase the wind on your body. p. 102

MT: MuscleTension Intervals; an on-the-bike resistance-training workout consisting of climbing hills at low cadences. pp. 103–104

OU: OverUnder Intervals; an interval workout during which you ride near your lactate threshold, increase intensity above it for a given time, and then reduce your intensity back to near-threshold. pp. 104–105

PI: PowerIntervals; a series of three-to-five-minute maximal intervals designed to increase your anaerobic power and your ability to repeat hard efforts with little recovery. pp. 105–106

PS: PowerStarts; an on-the-bike resistance-training workout targeted at your ATP/CP energy system. pp. 106–107

RS: RaceSimulation; a ride that closely resembles competition. Very often RS consists of a certain amount of time within a group ride. pp. 107–108

RR: RecoveryRide; one of the critical workouts for your success as a cyclist. These rides promote active recovery to better prepare your body for upcoming workouts. pp. 108–109

SI: SpeedIntervals; a series of short, high-cadence maximum efforts designed to increase your anaerobic power and repeatability. pp. 109–110

SS: SteadyState Intervals; one of the primary workouts for developing your sustainable power at lactate threshold. The length of the intervals, as well as the frequency of this workout within a week, leads to positive adaptation. pp. 110–111

S: Stomps; an on-the-bike resistance-training workout during which you accelerate a large gear (high initial resistance) while remaining seated. pp. 111–112

T: Tempo; one of the primary workouts for developing your ability to produce power aerobically. The long duration of this workout is what leads to positive adaptation. pp. 112–113

LT: Lactate Threshold; technically, the highest exercise-intensity level you can sustain before causing blood-lactate concentration to rise (more than 1 millimoles/liter) above exercise-baseline levels. Physiologically, LT is the point at which lactic acid accumulates faster than the body can clear and metabolize it. Practically, lactate threshold represents the highest power output you can sustain for prolonged (30- to 45-minute) periods of time.

VO$_2$max: a measure of an athlete's maximum oxygen consumption, and consequently a measure of an athlete's aerobic capacity. A high VO$_2$max is an indicator of high-endurance athletic potential, but not a guarantee of success.

Acknowledgments

Creating this book was made possible by spending the past thirty-plus years deeply involved in the sport of cycling. Many people played integral roles in my development as an athlete and coach, and hence in the creation of this book, and I am grateful to all of them.

I would like to thank Joe Avalos and Bill Woodul for giving me my first opportunities in cycling, as well as David Ware and Jack Nash for their invaluable support as I was learning to compete. I would also like to thank all the great cyclists on the 7-Eleven Team, whom I was fortunate enough to call my teammates, friends, and fellow pioneers.

Eddy Borysewicz, Jim Ochowicz, and Mike Neel were wonderful coaches in my years with the U.S. National Team and 7-Eleven, and they continue to be good friends. Many of the lessons they taught me have been vital to my development as a coach. Many thanks also to Jiri Mainus and all the coaches, mechanics, and staff members I worked with at USA Cycling. Their knowledge and commitment to excellence is unsurpassed in the world of athletics.

Of all the educators I had the pleasure of learning from, no other left as lasting an impression as Dr. Edmund Burke. Ed answered every question I ever asked him, and his impact on endurance sports will be felt for generations. Perhaps even more important than the advancements he made in human performance were the lessons he taught about communication and making information available for everyone. It is in that spirit that this book is dedicated to his memory.

I would like to thank all the people who make up Carmichael Training Systems for their dedication to making my vision a reality. Many of the CTS coaches played integral roles in putting this book together: Kathy Zawadzki contributed to the nutrition information in Chapter 7, Mike Niederpruem contributed to the physiology information in Chapters 4 and 5, and Erik Moen contributed his vast knowledge of bike fit in Chapter 6. You all are the very best, and we could not have achieved the things our company has without each and every one of you.

Of course, this section would be incomplete without thanking Lance Armstrong and all the athletes I have had the pleasure of coaching over the past thirteen years. I cannot imagine a career more fulfilling than this one.

To my mother and father, who were my first and always my best coaches, you have my eternal gratitude. The same is true for my brother and sister, who have always been there for me.

To my greatest joy, my family: Paige, Anna, and Connor, thank you for all your love and support. There is no greater experience in life than creating a family to share your years with.

Thank you to Susan Petersen Kennedy, Brian Tart, and Anna Cowles at Penguin for supporting this project from beginning to end.

And finally, a very special thank-you to Jim Rutberg, my friend and colleague. You are a man of many skills who continues to amaze me.

—*Chris Carmichael*

My thanks to Chris Carmichael for helping me reach my athletic and career goals, and to George Hincapie for introducing us. I would also like to thank the incredible group of coaches I have had the pleasure to learn from and work with: Jim Lehman, Craig Griffin, Dean Golich, Mike Niederpruem, Kathy Zawadzki, Erik Moen, James Herrera, Jason Koop, Ivana Bisaro, Daniel Gillespie, and Katie Compton. Thank you for helping to ensure that we didn't forget anything.

I also owe a debt of gratitude to all those who helped me gain the knowledge and experience to contribute to this book: Harry Havnoonian, Jim Alvord, and Paul Harrell for their support and coaching when I was a young athlete; Leslie Pearlman for her love, patience, and editing skills; and my family for always supporting my dreams.

Thank you to Brian Tart and Anna Cowles at Penguin, whose skilled and thoughtful editing was an essential and much appreciated part of bringing this book to print.

—*Jim Rutberg*

Index

Page numbers in *italic* indicate illustrations; those in **bold** indicate tables.

About the Authors

Chris Carmichael is a world-renowned cycling authority who has coached Tour de France Champion Lance Armstrong since 1990 and was inducted into the United States Bicycling Hall of Fame in May 2003. Part of the first American team to ride in the Tour de France, Carmichael was also a member of the 1984 U.S. Olympic Cycling Team. He served as the Men's Road Coach for the U.S. Olympic Cycling Team during the 1992 Olympic Games, and was the Head Coach for the U.S. Cycling Team for the 1996 Olympic Games. In 1999, he was awarded the prestigious U.S. Olympic Committee's Coach of the Year Award as well as the USA Cycling Coach of the Year Award. Athletes under his direction have won 33 Olympic, World Championship, and Pan American Game medals.

In 1999, he founded Carmichael Training Systems, Inc. (CTS, *www.train-right.com*) to share his coaching philosophy and methodology with cyclists and endurance athletes of all levels. A native of Miami, Florida, Carmichael and his wife, Paige, live in Colorado Springs with their two children, Anna and Connor.

Jim Rutberg has been a part of Carmichael Training Systems since its beginning. Originally as an athlete personally coached by Chris Carmichael and later as an employee, he learned the theory and practice of Carmichael Training Systems firsthand.

A cum laude graduate of Wake Forest University, Jim earned a Bachelor of Science degree in Health and Exercise Science. In addition to working as a coach, Jim's role at CTS has expanded into software development, content management, and business development. He has competed as a racing cyclist at the Elite National level throughout the United States. In 1999, he competed internationally at the Tour of Okinawa as a member of the U.S. National Cycling Team. A native of Philadelphia, Rutberg lives in Colorado Springs.

Questions for the authors? Email them at asktheauthor@trainright.com

Special Offer for *The Ultimate Ride* readers:

Get **ONE FREE* MONTH** of
Carmichael Training Systems Coaching!

To insure that *The Ultimate Ride* readers perform at their peak potential, CTS is providing readers with the following great offer for a limited time only.**

Your FREE* Excel CTS Coaching Program includes:
- Advice and guidance from CTS-Certified coaches
- Custom training program built around your specific schedule
- Training program based on *your* unique heart rate ranges

CTS Member Benefits:
- 10%-15% increase in power output
- Personal best race performance
- Greater results with less training time

How to get started with your FREE* coaching:
1. Sign up at **www.theultimateride.net**
2. Enter the special promotion code: theultimateride

That's it! It's easy. Start your coaching today!

Questions about this offer:
Email your questions to: **askcts@trainright.com**